4 April 2019

To Hannah

May you enjoy a career exclusively devoted to therapy!

Kavanaugh

HIPPOCRATES'
OATH
AND

ASCLEPIUS' SNAKE

HIPPOCRATES'

OATH

AND

ASCLEPIUS' SNAKE

The Birth of the Medical Profession

T.A. CAVANAUGH

OXFORD
UNIVERSITY PRESS

OXFORD
UNIVERSITY PRESS

Oxford University Press is a department of the University of Oxford. It furthers
the University's objective of excellence in research, scholarship, and education
by publishing worldwide. Oxford is a registered trade mark of Oxford University
Press in the UK and certain other countries.

Published in the United States of America by Oxford University Press
198 Madison Avenue, New York, NY 10016, United States of America.

Library of Congress Cataloging-in-Publication Data
Names: Cavanaugh, T. A., author.
Title: Hippocrates' oath and Asclepius' snake : the birth of the medical
profession / T.A. Cavanaugh.
Description: New York, NY: Oxford University Press, 2018. |
Includes bibliographical references and index.
Identifiers: LCCN 2017013746 (print) | LCCN 2017014393 (ebook) |
ISBN 9780190673680 (epub) | ISBN 9780190673697 (updf) |
ISBN 9780190673703 (online course) | ISBN 9780190673673 (cloth: alk. paper)
Subjects: | MESH: Hippocratic Oath
Classification: LCC R724.5 (ebook) | LCC R724.5 (print) | NLM W 50 |
DDC 174.2/2—dc23
LC record available at https://lccn.loc.gov/2017013746

9 8 7 6 5 4 3 2 1

Printed by Sheridan Books, Inc., United States of America

To Bonnie, my Beatrice, by whom gracious Lucy (*et alia*) illuminate *la diritta via*.

CONTENTS

ACKNOWLEDGMENTS

I thank my University of San Francisco students, colleagues, librarians, administrators, benefactors, and the faculty association. As a professor of philosophy, I enjoy many blessings that enable me to write a work such as this. These gifts include: first, the opportunity to teach; second, time to research and write; and third, material support that keeps body and soul together, stocks libraries with books, and enables me to travel (thanks to faculty development funds) to discuss ideas with others. I do not take these or the many other benefactions conferred on me as a member of the professoriate for granted. I hope this work evidences my gratitude and partially vindicates (although too feebly), among other wonders, my parents' (Thomas and Theresa) love of knowledge, my sisters' (Karen Inez, Julie Marie, and Mary Ann) sororal support, my own teachers' generosity, other parents' willingness to entrust the education of their offspring to faculty such as myself, and the generosity of myriad others supporting academia, whose groves I fortunately inhabit.

Proceeding alphabetically, I thank audiences at Baylor University, Brigham Young University's J. Reuben Clark School of Law, Catholic University of America's Columbus School of Law, Marquette University, Neumann University, the New University of Lisbon, the University of California (San Francisco), The University of Chicago, the University of Notre Dame, the University of Padova, and the University of Saint Thomas School of Law. To name names, I thank (for various assists with this and allied projects over the years, for any errors in which, of course, I answer): Professors Jason Eberl, Richard Fehring, Jorge Garcia, John Haldane, Thomas Hibbs, Joe Koterski, Edward Lyons, Steve McPhee, John O'Callaghan, David Solomon, Daniel Sulmasy, Lynn Wardle, and Joseph Zepeda. For her insightful editorial support, I thank Lucy Randall of OUP— thanks, too, to assistant editor Hannah Doyle. For his meticulous copyediting, I thank Steve Dodson. For her conscientious production editing, I thank Richa Jobin. For many kindnesses, many thanks to the Reverend C. M. Buckley, S.J. I thank my son Thomas Marcus Cavanaugh, who enthusiastically discussed homeopathy, among other topics. His love of truth (and a good fire with amenities) proves the enduring charm of a philosophic approach to knowledge and life more generally. I dedicate the work to my wife, Bonnie—*sine qua non* and the mistress of a constant attitude of gratitude.

HIPPOCRATES'
OATH
AND
ASCLEPIUS' SNAKE

INTRODUCTION

onsider this book's cover art. Today, one finds this Pentelic bas-relief sculpture in Naples's National Archeological Museum. Before Mt. Vesuvius's eruption (A.D. 79), one could have seen it in Herculaneum adorning a dwelling—now eponymously named after this masterpiece "the house of the Telephus relief." What goes on in the scene depicted? The viewer sees two intensely focused men. One stands while holding a knife and a spear to the abdomen of the other, seated. While the points of both weapons impress upon the man, they—just barely—do not pierce him. Certainly, they retain their menacing character. No one would opt to be the seated man. Tension permeates the encounter.

Here, we witness the legendary healing of Telephus by Achilles (treated extensively in chapter 1). With his knife, Achilles scrapes filings from his spear (with which he had previously wounded him) into Telephus' long-festering wound. Prior to the therapy pictured, the Delphic oracle tells a desperate cure-seeking Telephus that only the wounder can heal him. With the very weapon with which he injured him, Achilles does. As the oracle states, the wounder heals. This pithy truth (which, in 1.1, I refer to as the homeopathic principle) points to an allied, more worrisome phenomenon. Namely, just as the wounder heals, so too does the healer wound—the problem of iatrogenic harm. In Greek, *iatros* and *genos* mean "doctor" and "born of," respectively. Hence, an iatrogenic wound is one attributed to a physician. Such wounds take three salient forms: wounds ineliminable from therapy, such as cauterizing to stop bleeding; harmful errors committed while caregiving, such as administering the wrong dose of a drug; and, last of all, what I call wounds of role-conflation, such as euthanizing a patient or assisting his suicide (at his request). In the last type of wound (the most problematic), a physician adopts the role of wounder by deliberately injuring, thereby abandoning the practice of medicine as an exclusively therapeutic activity.

I argue that the Hippocratic *Oath* (articulated in chapter 2), which incorporates both a contract (concerning the novel teaching of the medical art to unrelated males, explicated in 2.2.2) and an oath-proper (which deals with a physician's interactions with patients, treated of in 2.2.3), responds to the profound threat role-conflation poses to medical practice. By means of the *Oath*, Hippocrates (whom I regard as its author, for reasons enunciated in 2.1) founds medicine as a profession devoted wholly to therapy, explicitly excluding deliberate wounding. Having closely examined the *Oath* in chapter 2, I argue on behalf of it in chapter 3, especially for its contention (found in the oath-proper) that a physician electively killing a patient, even at the request of that patient, instances harm and injustice. In chapter 3, I advance numerous reasons for regarding a doctor's involvement in killing as a profound error that entirely disorients medicine as an exclusively therapeutic practice. Further, I advance the *Oath's* implicit claim that iatrogenic harm (especially in the form of role-conflation as instanced by, e.g., Dr. Guillotin, whose example serves in chapter 3 as a cautionary tale) amounts to the foundational medical-ethical problem, the answer to which (found in the *Oath*) inaugurates medicine as a profession (in contrast to, e.g., conflicts of interest being medicine's basic moral issue).

In chapter 4 (the final chapter), I examine the intimate connections between medicine as incorporating an oath, being a profession, and possessing autonomy. I argue that professional medical practice cannot amount solely to a technique. Rather, it necessarily incorporates an internal medical ethic, to which practitioners swear. In chapter 4, I argue that the most basic indisputable norm internal to medical practice approximates the pithy aphorism found in *Epidemics* (I, 11), "as to diseases, practice two: help or do not harm" (Hippocrates, 1962, 164–5, author's translation). Or, to employ a more familiar Latin saying (whose exact origins remain obscure but may be bound up with *Epidemics* I, 11, as noted in 1.2): *primum, non nocere*—"first, do no harm."

I conclude chapter 4 by noting that medical oath-taking, e.g., in the White Coat Ceremony, is enjoying a renaissance. Accordingly, the implications of medical promising—including self-regulation, public education, and societal respect for professional conscientious objection to requests for interventions incompatible with one's promise (treated in 4.3)—deserve increased attention. The appendix presents the Greek text of the *Oath* and a literal English translation.

At this juncture, two overarching questions arise: "What?" and "So what?" Briefly (and in answer to the first question), I present what follows as a work in medical ethics that relies on contributions from numerous disciplines, including history, classics, and philosophy. Having articulated the *Oath*, I argue on behalf of the ethical commitments the juror makes to the sick (the oath-proper). One finds the principal contribution here, in the argument for a conception of medicine as inherently therapeutic, excluding injuring. This, of course, brings us to our second question: "So what?"

What relevance, if any, does a medical ethic dating to around the middle of the fifth century B.C. have for our times? Lest I be misunderstood at the outset, I do not propose that the *Oath* can serve as an ethical cure-all—or, to use a word found in the *Oath* itself, a panacea. Needless to say, it does not have all the answers we seek. Rather, as I will argue in what follows, the *Oath* establishes boundaries within which ethical medicine takes place. The establishment of limits within which to practice medicine has critical importance. For (as I argue in 4.2) boundaries further a practice's flourishing. Concerning such matters, the *Oath* reasonably, practically, and succinctly answers questions a medical practitioner in any age must address. Most broadly, it answers what one will do with the medical art (benefit the sick) and what one will not do with it (deliberately injure). With respect to the latter, the *Oath* specifies certain still salient injuries not to be visited upon a patient, such as giving a deadly drug. I argue on behalf of the *Oath's* judgment that such an injury is to be avoided (for numerous reasons) in professional medical practice. In part because questions concerning the compatibility (or lack thereof) of killing with medicine as a profession continue to confront us, the *Oath* signally merits our attention. The ease with which one can refer to medicine as a profession points to another aspect of the *Oath's* lasting relevance—namely, medicine as involving a profession.

As a practice, medicine (roughly) has a discernible point of departure. As is the case with many contemporary practices (to name a few: physics, tragedy, comedy, philosophy, economics, and politics—all of whose names derive from the Greek language), we find medicine's genesis in the Ancient Greek world. Coincident with that beginning one finds the *Oath*. The *Oath* embodies a conception of medical practice as intimately involving a profession about what one will and will not do (a medical ethic) with one's technical expertise. Thus, one finds part of the *Oath's* legacy in our robust intuitive sense that medicine, a paradigmatic profession, appropriately involves promising.

Finally, to take but one of countless works from antiquity, Sophocles' *Oedipus the Tyrant* continues to enlighten us, for the human condition has timeless aspects about which the ancient tragedy still speaks insightfully. Similarly, the *Oath* illuminates the therapeutic path. Accordingly, let us turn to Hippocrates' *Oath* and Asclepius' Snake.

Chapter 1
SNAKE?

1.1 ASCLEPIUS' SNAKE

Asclepius' snake—a single serpent wrapped about a walking staff—indicates our need for Hippocrates' *Oath*. For, as I will argue, this snake symbolic of the healing profession prompts a basic question the answer to which founds what we have come to call medicine. As posed to the snake, the question would be: "do you bite?" As asked of the physician: "do you wound?" Our investigation begins with this ancient medical symbol as revelatory of this vexing ethical question, to which the author of the *Oath* emphatically answers, "No." (For the time being and without argument, I refer to Hippocrates as the author of the *Oath*. In chapter 2, I offer reasons for so speaking.)

Consider the intriguing connection between medicine and snakes. We see snakes depicted on hospitals, ambulances, medical equipment, and physicians' white coats. We take such images for granted, hardly remarking upon them. If we pause and think about them, however, such symbols should perplex us. Typically, we understand serpents to be vile, dangerous, and venomous; many find them, literally, creepy. Moreover, snakes wound. Why employ them to depict healing? They seem more suited to represent soldiers than physicians.

In what follows, I argue that snakes precisely as wounders paradoxically yet aptly symbolize physicians and medicine more generally. Attending to the snake as medicine's symbol enables us to think more clearly about the nature of medicine and the unique defining problem perennially confronting its practitioners: that of ridding healing of wounding. Moreover, understanding the appropriateness of the snake as the symbol of medicine illuminates the import of the Hippocratic *Oath*. This, however, is to get ahead of ourselves. Let us first consider the two different snake-themed images competing to represent medicine.

First, imagine two snakes entwining a wand. We call this symbol the caduceus. Second, conjure up the aforementioned rough-hewn wooden staff with one snake wrapping itself around it: the rod of Asclepius. Consider the caduceus first. You have, no doubt, encountered this image, maybe on an ambulance or in a pharmacy. In the early 1900s, one would have seen it on the new offices of the American Medical Association in Chicago. Since 1902, it has served as the insignia of the US Army Medical Corps. A ubiquitous emblem of healing, it is found on numerous medical school buildings and hospitals, as well as in doctor's offices. Physicians and nurses come across it frequently in their daily practice, whether on medical equipment or pharmaceutical advertising. As omnipresent as the caduceus is, and as frequently as it is offered and accepted as a medical logo, it is not a historically accurate symbol of medicine. Rather, it is the rod of the Greek god Hermes (the Roman god Mercury), who, after Homer's usage, comes to be called the *kērux* or messenger of the gods. We do not know the origins of the caduceus with any precision.[1] We do know that the Greek word *kērux* (herald or public messenger) gives rise to *kērukeion*, which means "herald's staff," which in turn, by the twists and turns which change language, leads to the Latin *caduceus*, the term we use today.

As messenger of the gods, Hermes bears the original rod from which we derive the staff topped with two snakes. Precisely how the snakes become affixed remains lost in the mists of history. Some myths suggest that during a mission for the gods, Hermes encountered two snakes fighting or, perhaps, copulating. He cast his rod into their midst. They twisted themselves around it; they have been there ever since. Whatever the case may be, we do know that in antiquity messengers carried distinct rods (without snakes) in order to identify themselves as envoys and thereby to enjoy the unique protections afforded them, such as immunity from attack and protection in alien lands. Thus, Hermes carries such a rod as messenger of the gods.[2] Among other roles, Hermes also serves as the deity of thieves and conductor of the dead to Hades; hardly a good icon for physicians. How did his caduceus become associated with medicine?

In *The Golden Wand of Medicine*, the medical humanist, professor of neurology, and physician Walter Friedlander presents the tale of how, particularly in the United States, the medical community mistook the caduceus for the historically accurate medical symbol, the (soon to be discussed) one-snake rod of Asclepius. To recount that story briefly, in the early 1500s the relatively new profession of printing (originating around 1455 with the first Gutenberg Bible) was seeking a symbol by which to represent itself.[3] Because Hermes was the messenger of the gods, printers—casting themselves in the role of important messengers—hit upon the caduceus as their trademark. Thus, in Europe, the caduceus became a standard printer's mark. Three hundred years later, in the United States, it became associated with medicine. It did so in part because one of the chief medical textbook publishers for the US market, Churchill of London, employed the caduceus liberally on the title pages of medical textbooks published in the 1840s. As Friedlander notes, while Churchill himself clearly understood the caduceus to be the mark of his trade as a publisher, some among his US audience of professors and students of medicine, knowing vaguely that the medical symbol involved a rod and snake, mistook the two-snake rod to be the proper sign of medicine.[4] Indeed, within forty years of the introduction of Churchill's volumes, US publishers of medical textbooks adopted the caduceus, not as a printer's mark but, rather, as the symbol of medicine. Now, let us put the caduceus to the side in order to consider the correct icon of medicine.

To imagine the historically accurate symbol of medicine, we must picture our second image, the noted staff of Asclepius, a rough-hewn wooden rod with one snake entwined about it. Asclepius is the Greek demigod of medicine. We first hear of him—twice referred to as the "blameless physician" (*amumonos iētēros*) —in Homer's *Iliad* (iv, line 194, Homer 1999b, 178; xi, line 518, 530). Notably, Asclepius' rod differs from Hermes' as a walking-stick differs from a wand. The walking-staff reflects the itinerant character of the Ancient Greek doctor. A physician went from one village to another on foot. Indeed, "epidemiology" (the name of the discipline that studies the spread of disease) derives from the Greek *epi* (about) and *dēmos* (village). In the Hippocratic corpus, the volumes entitled *Epidemics* concern not the spread of disease but, rather, the different medical cases the physician encounters as he walks from one village to another. Accordingly, Asclepius' staff represents the walking stick a physician would employ. This, of course, does not account for the snake. Why associate a snake with medicine? Why does the reptile coil itself about Asclepius' staff? Although this is initially puzzling, a number of reasons suggest the appropriateness of symbolizing medicine by a snake. Consider the following.

First, snakes exemplify one of the most dramatic forms of molting (called ecdysis), in which a creature sheds its entire covering at once. While other animals shed feathers, fur, and skin a little at a time, snakes discard their skins in one fell swoop, leaving an intact, inverted sloughed-off skin, or exuviae. This remarkable characteristic understandably gives rise to the impression that snakes have the ability to heal and renew themselves. Thus, they serve as a fit symbol for healing more generally.

Second, snakes are understandably regarded as possessing an intimate familiarity with the earth. Typically, they spend their lives entirely on and in the earth. Most snakes do not rise above the ground, but remain always in contact with it. Given their constant proximity to the earth, snakes aptly symbolize an intimate, rare, hard-to-acquire knowledge of the earth's hidden healing properties, found, for instance, in minerals and herbs. As earthly creatures, snakes aptly represent medicine as a wisdom concerning the earth's healing properties.

Historians of medicine propose a third possible reason for the association of snakes with medicine. They note that in Africa, the Arabian Peninsula, and Asia, we find a parasite called *Dracunculus medinensis* (literally, "little dragon of Medina"). This parasite causes the illness named *dracunculiasis*, a Latin term meaning "afflicted with little dragons," also known as guinea-worm disease. The parasite derives the latter part of its name (*medinensis*) from the (present-day) Saudi Arabian city of Medina, as the infestation was so common there in antiquity. One of the oldest documented parasitic illnesses, records of guinea-worm disease date back 2,000 years before Christ. The disease is contracted by ingesting the larvae of the parasite in contaminated drinking water. Once inside the victim, the larvae hatch and mate. The fertilized female worm then descends to one of the feet of the victim, where she emerges from the skin. The ancient treatment for this disease—and one still employed in developing countries—is to take a slender stick and place it at the exit wound so that the worm will wrap herself about the stick. Some medical historians propose that the snake-like creature wrapped about what has come to be considered Asclepius' walking-rod actually represents a guinea worm entwined about a stick. They hypothesize that ancient physicians advertised themselves by means of this symbol. As the Italians might remark, "*se non è vero, è ben trovato,*" or, loosely translated, "even if it is not true, at least it makes for a good story."

Medical historians get a lot of mileage out of the humble guinea worm. Some suggest that one striking instance in which a snake comes to symbolize healing may refer to guinea-worm disease. Recall the following story from the *Pentateuch*:

And they journeyed from mount Hor by the way of the Red sea, to compass the land of Edom: and the soul of the people was much discouraged because of the way. And the people spake against God, and against Moses, Wherefore have ye brought us up out of Egypt to die in the wilderness? for there is no bread, neither is there any water; and our soul loatheth this light bread. And the Lord sent fiery serpents among the people, and they bit the people; and much people of Israel died. Therefore the people came to Moses, and said, We have sinned, for we have spoken against the Lord, and against thee; pray unto the Lord, that he take away the serpents from us. And Moses prayed for the people. And the Lord said unto Moses, Make thee a fiery serpent, and set it upon a pole: and it shall come to pass, that every one that is bitten, when he looketh upon it, shall live. And Moses made a serpent of brass, and put it upon a pole, and it came to pass, that if a serpent had bitten any man, when he beheld the serpent of brass, he lived. (Numbers 21:4–9, King James Version)

Perhaps the Israelites had been afflicted with the indigenous guinea worm? Regardless, here we see the very being which wounds taken as the symbol of healing. Indeed, even more remarkably, the snake-symbol actually heals. Moreover, this occurs in a culture in which the snake, as found in *Genesis*, exemplifies a wounder.

The above instance of the snake's association with healing becomes even more noteworthy upon Jesus' reference to it, found in John's gospel:

And as Moses lifted up the serpent in the wilderness, even so
must the Son of man be lifted up: That whosoever believeth
in him should not perish, but have eternal life. (John 3:14–15,
King James Version)

Thus, Jesus compares himself lifted up on the cross to Moses' bronze
serpent; just as those who looked upon the bronze serpent were physically healed, so shall those who believe in the crucified Jesus be healed
spiritually. Hence, to take three salient instances, we see pagan Greeks,
ancient Jews, and early Christians using the snake as a symbol for (and
even a cause of) healing.

This brings me to the fourth, final, and, for our purposes, most
significant reason for symbolizing medicine with a snake. I call it the
"like cures like" reason, or, in medical terms, the homeopathic principle.
Snakes well represent medicine because a basic (and ancient) medical
insight is that the cause of a wound at times also heals. Or, as the Greeks
via the Delphic oracle put it (as we shall see shortly): the wounder
heals. I propose that reflection on this paradoxical truth of medical
therapy leads to the oldest extant medical ethic, the Hippocratic *Oath*.
That is (as I will argue in the next chapter), the *Oath* responds to the
intimate relation between healing and wounding. But this is to get
slightly ahead of myself.

At this point, I hope to establish that while we understandably find it
perplexing that the snake—that venomous, viperous, literally creepy creature ("serpent" comes from the Latin *serpere*, which means to creep)—
symbolizes healing, it makes sense that a paradigmatic wounder would

serve as the image of healing. For, as the homeopathic insight shows us, the wounder heals. Allow me, then, to offer evidence for this claim.

Numerous medical traditions—including the Hippocratic writings[5]— propose that "like cures like," the homeopathic principle.[6] "Homeo-" is from Greek *homoios*, which means "similar," and "-pathic" is from Greek *pathos*, meaning "suffering, disease"; thus, "homeopathic" means "similar to the disease." Briefly, the homeopathic principle can be construed in a more general, noncontroversial manner or in a much more specific (and controverted) fashion. In its most general form, the homeopathic principle would simply have one treat a patient suffering from a disease that produces, for example, heat as a symptom (say a fever) with something hot (rather than something cold). The homeopathic principle in its more specific (and disputed) formulation derives from the occasionally noted phenomenon that substances that in healthy people induce symptoms like those caused by an illness at times cure sick people of that very illness.[7] With this phenomenon in mind, the German physician Samuel Hahnemann coins the term *Homöopathie* (from which we get "homeopathy") in 1807.[8] Like cures like. That which produces in healthy people symptoms similar to those of a specific sickness sometimes restores health in those who suffer from that ailment. Hence, the homeopath proposes to treat the sick with that therapy. Lest I be misunderstood as an advocate, I do not propose or endorse an overarching homeopathic approach to medical practice—as, for example, Hahnemann does. Rather, I note that an ancient practice-based observation (homeopathy) has deeper implications, to which I now turn.

Given their love of paradox (found in their pithy command "know thyself" —how could one fail in this apparently easy task?), the conjunction of wounding with healing struck the Greeks with particular force. Indeed, one finds the wounder healing at the heart of a famous legend dramatized by each of the greatest tragedians: Aeschylus, Sophocles, and Euripides. Unfortunately, only fragments of the relevant plays survive, the greatest number by far coming from Euripides' tragedy.

In March of 438 B.C., Euripides offered *Telephus* to the Athenians. He did so in the annual Great Dionysia, a religious festival to Dionysius, the god of wine. Fortunately for us, but painfully for Euripides, in the audience there may have been a precocious youth named Aristophanes, who would go on to become the greatest writer of Greek comedies. We are lucky that, whether or not he was present, he acquired an intimate knowledge of and apparent fascination with the play. (Of his numerous references to Euripides, this play has the largest number; it impressed itself upon him.) For it is primarily through him that we know this otherwise lost tragedy. Euripides, however, has less reason to thank Aristophanes. Thirteen years later, in his comedy *Acharnians*, Aristophanes went on to mercilessly parody the drama he presumably witnessed that day. Indeed, Aristophanes seems never to tire of parodying Euripides' *Telephus*. We find him lampooning it even in his last extant comedy, *Plutus*. (We also owe a debt of gratitude to Aristophanes for *Plutus*, from which, as will become more evident in 2.2.1, we receive our most complete description of the healing rituals employed in an Asclepion—a temple to Asclepius, the noted Greek demigod of healing.)

Relying on fragments from or concerning Delphic oracular statements, Euripides' *Telephus*, Aristophanes' caricatures of the same, and various other sources, one can (albeit roughly) limn Telephus' story as follows. In their first (and unsuccessful) expedition to attack Troy, the Greeks assault Telephus' kingdom, mistaking it for Troy. Telephus mounts a successful defense, but Achilles wounds him. The Greeks depart. Telephus' wound festers; no physician can heal it. (Notably, wounds that fester come to be called "telephian".)[9] At wit's end, Telephus consults the oracle of Apollo (the god of healing) at Delphi, asking "what is the remedy?" (Fontenrose 1978, 368–9). The oracle advises him that "the wounder will heal" (*ho trōsas iasetai* (Parke and Wormell 1961, 83). Puzzled, Telephus goes to Argos, where the Greeks are assembling for a second attack upon Troy. He hopes that Achilles will restore him to health. Asked to treat Telephus, Achilles responds that he is not a healer. The wise Ulysses realizes that Apollo-physician does not mean that Achilles will mend Telephus. Rather, Achilles' spear—or as it actually turns out, Achilles and his spear—will cure Telephus. Achilles scrapes filings from his spear into Telephus' festering wound (as depicted on this book's cover). Telephus is healed. Accordingly, along with the aforementioned reasons for associating the snake with medicine, we have the homeopathic principle. Or, as the oracle paradoxically states: "the wounder heals." Thus, precisely in its role as wounder the snake aptly serves as a symbol of the healer.

1.2 IATROGENIC HARM

In light of the wounder healing, I make a simple claim; namely, that insofar as the wounder heals, it is also true—indeed, to that very extent true—that the healer wounds. Again, consider Euripides' *Telephus*. The oracle tells us that the wounder heals. All the characters and we the audience attend to this, for it is the puzzle upon which Euripides focuses our attention. Achilles (and his spear) who wounded Telephus becomes a healer while also remaining a wounder. That is, there is a mirror image, flip side, corresponding paradox, or isomorph to the homeopathic principle: the healer wounds. Let us call this fact that the healer wounds the iatrogenic problem. We derive the word "iatrogenic" from the Greek *iatros* "physician" and *genos* "born of." As the Greek etymology indicates, a physician causes an iatrogenic disease. While the wounder's healing (the homeopathic principle) does not prove ethically problematic—indeed, we find a wounder's healing wonderful—the healer's wounding (the iatrogenic conundrum) certainly does. A healer's wounding naturally troubles us. Indeed, in the Hippocratic corpus we encounter the aphoristic rule of medical practice that one should "at least, do no harm," which appears at some point to have been Latinized as "*primum, non nocere*," better known in its English translation as "first, do no harm."[10] Clearly, a concern to avoid wounding one's patient looms large from the very beginnings of reflection upon medical practice.

Briefly, how does the healer wound? Consider three kinds of wounds a healer inflicts. The first I will call wounds of treatment (or therapy); the second, errors; and the third, for lack of a better phrase, I will call role-conflation, to refer to the healer deliberately adopting the role of wounder. The Hippocratic *Oath* addresses all three, singling out for special attention that of role-conflation.

First, consider wounds of treatment. Wounds of treatment include cutting, stitching, cauterizing, sticking with needles, drugging, and myriad complications such as blood clots that occasionally attend medical therapies. While one can reduce treatment-wounds such as incisions by making them smaller, less conspicuous, and less enduring, one cannot eliminate them from the practice of medicine, for healing involves cutting, burning, drugging, and subjecting patients to the complications of medical treatment.

When it comes to drugs, we commonly speak of these wounds as "side effects," a useful phrase as long as we realize that in so naming their deleterious effects, we thereby incorporate a judgment about intent. That is, although the oncologist in fact poisons his patient, we call his act one of therapy because he intends those aspects of the poison that kill cancer and not those aspects of the poison that sicken his patient. One might understandably regard this as so obvious as not to merit comment. Of course, the nausea, debilitation, and susceptibility to infection caused by the chemotherapy are side effects. The oncologist administers the drug to kill cancer, not to cause these foreseen outcomes. I draw the distinction between what physicians intend and what they foresee but do not intend to simply note how crucial and taken-for-granted such an observation remains to the daily practice of medicine. (We will return to this and allied considerations in 3.5 and 4.3.2, when we address harms foreseen but not intended by the physician insofar as they concomitantly attend therapy.) Again, while these wounds of cutting, burning, and drugging can be reduced, they cannot be eliminated from medicine. They remain part and parcel of good, even excellent medical practice. Yet, why would this be so? Why not think that medicine could become free of treatment-wounds?

An adequate answer to that question would amount to a study in itself. However, the above claim that such wounds attend even very good doctoring requires elaboration. Briefly, dis-ease instances disorder of the body. To remedy disease (using that term broadly), one must re-establish the body's order, health. The acts of re-establishing health (heating or cooling, bandaging cuts and removing bandages, administering drugs, and so on) themselves have obnoxious aspects insofar as they necessarily involve moving the body from a state of disease to a state of health. The disagreeable aspects, of course, instance treatment-wounds. They amount to the friction (as it were) encountered in movement. To take but one of myriad instances, consider the setting of a broken nose. A broken nose is crooked. To remedy it, one must straighten it. To do so, one must rebreak it. Hence, a broken nose requires breaking. Breaking, bleeding, and subsequent swelling cannot be avoided in the setting of a nose. It—as would countless other examples—illustrates ineliminable treatment-wounds that attend sound medical practice. Now, consider errors.

Harmful errors comprise the second class of wounds associated with medicine. Medicine is and will always remain a human enterprise.

To err is human. Thus, error—sometimes harmful—attends medicine. Unlike a treatment-wound, however, a harmful error, to be an error, must be defective and avoidable. Thus, error is a falling away from good medical practice. This distinguishes ineliminable wounds of treatment from avoidable wounds of error. The avoidability of error, however, suggests that there could be such a thing as error-free medicine. This further suggests that "to err is human" might not apply to the medical forum. Perhaps the fallibility attending ordinary humans could be overcome in medicine? To the contrary, while it is true to say of any error that it could have been avoided, since medicine will always remain a practice of humans, error will always attend medicine. For medicine remains, and always will remain, an empirical, experiential activity. Thus, we will constantly be discovering what kinds of mistakes we make. One fruitful response to medical error is to recognize that something has gone wrong and the individual practitioner is at fault, while also noting that the mistake of this one practitioner may very well reveal to the entire body of practitioners an error to be avoided.[11]

Allow me to illustrate using a pedestrian medication error:

[A concerned individual] alerted investigators participating in a study of ... [a drug] ... of a problem related to product concentration. The [pharmaceutical] company had received reports of users who had read the label on the 5-mL container, also saw the concentration (10 mg/mL), and concluded that the entire container held 10 mg. The volume did

> appear on the label, but these users did not see it. Three
> patients received a fivefold overdose of [the drug] ... and
> one patient died. The product is now on the market with an
> improved label. (Cohen 1999, 13.10)

The author notes precisely the same problem with similar fatal results for other drugs in which the volume and the strength of the dose were not adequately labeled. While the system of labeling set the caregiver up to make this mistake, it is still true that the caregiver erred. The erring physician failed in this instance in the practice of his art, as all artists do, be they doctors, musicians, or professors.

I have claimed that there are at least three kinds of wounds illustrative of the healer's wounding; namely, wounds of treatment, wounds of error, and wounds of role-conflation. It is to this third and final type that I now turn. I propose that his recognition of iatrogenic harm, especially as found in the wounds of role-conflation, prompted Hippocrates to compose the *Oath*.

1.3 THE MEDICAL-ETHICAL PROBLEM: ROLE-CONFLATION

The *Oath* begins, "I swear by Apollo, physician, and Asclepius, and Hygieia and Panaceia and all the gods and goddesses ..." Note that the oath-taker swears by "Apollo, physician," while he does not specify the role of the other gods and goddesses. He does so in part because Apollo occupies a number of disparate roles. In addition to being the god of healing, he is the god of music, of assemblies, of prophecy, of the sun, and, more importantly for our purposes, of plague and disease. It is upon this last role that I want to focus. For as the god of both healing and of sickening, Apollo suggests the difficulty facing Hippocrates: namely, the need to exclude the role of wounder from that of healer.

We find one striking portrayal of Apollo as a wounder in Homer's *Iliad*. At the beginning of the epic, Homer tells us that Apollo spreads plague among the Greeks in answer to the prayers of his priest Chryses, whose daughter Chryseis had been taken by Agamemnon, the leader of the Greeks. The god of healing is also the god of sickening. Indeed, the priest Chryses prays precisely for Apollo to visit a pestilence upon the Greeks. What is the import of this? Clearly, it instances the iatrogenic problem: Apollo, physician, also wounds. Indeed, just as he heals in response to prayers and supplications, so also he injures at the request of a beloved petitioner. This harming, however, does not occur incidentally to healing. It is neither a treatment-wound nor an error. Rather, Apollo deliberately wounds. He chooses to afflict. By electing to spread disease among the Greeks, Apollo-healer illustrates role-conflation.

Another instance of wounding via role-conflation concerns Asclepius, the demigod of healing subordinate to Apollo (his father) by whom Hippocrates also swears. Asclepius occupies fewer roles than Apollo. However, he, like Apollo, both heals and wounds. Indeed, among the myths concerning Asclepius one tells us that from Medusa he received two vials of blood, one from her right side and one from her left. With the vial of blood from her right side, he healed; with the vial of blood from her left side, he sickened. He, as does Apollo, stands indeterminately toward the ends of healing and sickening and, correspondingly, the roles of healer and wounder. Apollo and Asclepius both play these opposed roles deliberately, employing one art ambivalently to produce health or sickness.

Call this indeterminacy regarding the end on behalf of which one uses the technique the Apollonian-Asclepian view of medicine. (For the time being I treat the Apollonian-Asclepian account as monolithic. Later, in 3.1 I distinguish the Apollonian from the Asclepian practice in terms of how they diversely incorporate killing.) In this approach, the medical art has the character solely of a technique, a know-how or skill that can be ordered toward opposing goals while itself remaining the same. Thus, to take an extreme example, consider a physician administering capital punishment by means of a lethal injection. From the Apollonian-Asclepian perspective, this act makes perfect sense. After all, who can execute as well as a physician? Who can kill more humanely than the healer? Lest one think this example fanciful, recall (as we will discuss at greater length in 3.3.2) that the guillotine derives its name from Guillotin, a physician, its most reputable and famous advocate. As Socrates in Plato's *Republic* notes:

> [Socrates:] Who then is the most able when they are ill to benefit friends and harm enemies in respect to disease and health?
>
> [Polemarchus:] The physician. (Plato 1961, 332d-4, 581-2)

Why can the physician so benefit friends and harm enemies? Consider this insight from Plato's student, Aristotle, found in his *Metaphysics*:

> Hence all arts [*technai*], *i.e.* the productive sciences, are potencies; because they are principles of change in another thing, or in the artist himself *qua* [as] other. Every rational potency admits equally of contrary results, but irrational potencies admit of one result only. *E.g.*, heat can only produce heat, but medical science [*iatrikē*, the productive medical science or art] can produce disease and health. The reason of this is that science [*epistēmē*] is a rational account, and the same account explains both the thing and its privation, though not in the same way. (Aristotle 1989, 1046b4–9, 432–3)

Health is ease; illness is the lack of health, dis-ease. Knowledge of how to foster health naturally includes knowledge of how to produce sickness. Thus, the practitioner can further illness or health.

Indeed, the more virtuoso, the more capable of facilitating either. As Aristotle notes in the *Nicomachean Ethics*, "in art [*technē*] one who errs voluntarily is preferable" (Aristotle 1990a, 1140b23–24, 338, author's translation). An artist displays virtuosity by producing either of the opposed effects in question. The best orator can produce both belief and disbelief; the best architect can produce symmetry and asymmetry; the best physician can produce health and sickness. Again, to know how to produce the one, be it persuasion, symmetry, or health, confers knowledge about how to produce its privation. Technique itself stands ambivalent between opposites; so, too, does the technician as technician.

Yet one might think it clearly and emphatically false that the best physician also makes, for example, the best poisoner or executioner. For, as a type, the physician does not poison or execute. Indeed, by the reckoning of many (including, of course, Hippocrates), the healer who poisons no longer merits the name. To take but one such thinker, again consider what Aristotle (whose father was a doctor) says in the *Nicomachean Ethics*:

> We deliberate not about ends, but about means toward the end. For the physician does not deliberate about if he will heal, nor the rhetorician about if he will persuade, nor the politician about if he will make good order, nor do any of the rest deliberate about his end. But laying down some end, we examine how and through what it comes to be. (Aristotle 1990a, 1112b12–17, author's translation)[12]

This text suggests that excellent physicians, rhetoricians, and politicians deliberately and exclusively heal, persuade, and make good order. The politician does not choose to make bad government. The rhetorician does not elect to make specious arguments. Similarly, the physician does not try to sicken. For each, to paraphrase Aristotle, has already laid down some end. Thus, they now "examine how and through what it comes to be." Therefore, when we speak of a physician, we speak of one who has made a determination (from the Latin, *terminare*, meaning "to mark the end," the terminus) that he will heal, exclusively. Accordingly, those who have the goal of healing do not poison, for to do so would be to betray the end laid down. Indeed, it would amount to adopting an objective diametrically opposed to and contradictory of healing, the goal which defines the physician. As I will argue (in 2.2.3), the *Oath* definitively lays down this end. Prior to this determination, however, the Apollonian-Asclepian view appears viable.

To reflect further on the laying down of ends, consider how the sophist differs from the orator. We distinguish the duo while acknowledging that both possess the same competence, skill, technique, or art, as Aristotle indicates:

> It is a function of one and the same art to see the persuasive and [to see] the apparently persuasive, just as [it is] in dialectic [to recognize] a syllogism and [to recognize] an apparent syllogism; for sophistry is not a matter of ability [*dynamis*] but of deliberate choice [*prohairesis*] [of specious arguments]. In the case of rhetoric, however, there is the difference that one person will be [called] *rhetor* on the basis of his knowledge [*episteme*] and another on the basis of his deliberative choice, while in dialectic sophist refers to deliberative choice [of specious arguments], dialectician not to deliberate choice, but to ability [at argument generally].[13]

The rhetorician and the sophist both know how to move audiences by speech. They do not differ in this respect; rather, they differ in their choices concerning both by what means and to what ends they will use this shared skill. Orators will not use specious arguments. Moreover, they will move their audience toward what they apprehend as true. Sophists, by contrast, will use deceptive arguments. Moreover, they will move their audience, willy-nilly, to embrace what they consider true or false conclusions. Similarly, the physician and the poisoner do not differ in their knowledge of drugs. Rather, they differ in the choices they make concerning to what ends they will put their knowledge of drugs to use: the one to heal, the other to sicken—even, perhaps, to kill.

This difference in choice between the mender and the render poses a number of problems. Consider a few. Given their technical similarity, how does one differentiate the healer from the wounder? How does the physician who practices the medical art as duly ordered only toward healing communicate this to patients, peers, prospective students, and the public more generally? How does a patient who seeks the aid of one devoted exclusively to healing discern that a practitioner has definitively chosen to heal and not to sicken? How does a student who wants to learn this art so understood find such a teacher? How does the public identify those who propose to practice medicine solely as therapeutic?

The choice confronting the possessor of the ambivalent (healing/ wounding) technique constitutes the inaugural medical-ethical issue, the decision concerning which profoundly defines medicine. For it determines what the practitioner will pursue as his end. Those who seek caregivers devoted exclusively to healing (peer-practitioners, patients, prospective students, and the public more generally) need those who practice to stand before them and tell them what they stand for, what they have as their goal. Literally, they need doctors to make a profession. Hippocrates' *Oath* meets precisely this need. With it, the possessor of the skill that can both heal and sicken pledges only to heal. The capacity to sicken will always remain, for it belongs to the technique. By the juror's professed determination, however, the physician rejects that possible use of the art.

Aware of the iatrogenic problem, Hippocrates aspires to eradicate deliberate wounding from the healer's role by means of the *Oath*. This hope—informed by Greek myth, tragedy, and medical practice—serves as one of the chief motives for recourse to a sacred oath. Commenting on the Hippocratic *Oath*, the anthropologist Margaret Mead says:

> For the first time in our tradition there was a complete separation between killing and curing. Throughout the primitive world the doctor and the sorcerer tended to be the same person. He with power to kill had power to cure, including specially the undoing of his own killing activities. He who had power to cure would necessarily also be able to kill. With the Greeks, ... the distinction was made clear. One profession ... [was] to be dedicated completely to life under all circumstances, regardless of rank, age, or intellect—the life of a slave, the life of the Emperor, the life of a foreign man, the life of a defective child. ... this is a priceless possession which we cannot afford to tarnish, but society is always attempting to make the physician into a killer—to kill the defective child at birth, to leave the sleeping pills beside the bed of the cancer patient ... it is the duty of society to protect the physician from such requests. (Levine 1972, 324–5)[14]

Hippocrates cannot rid medicine of all wounding. As noted, treatment-wounds attend excellent medical practice, while error accompanies medicine as an activity of fallible humans. Accordingly, these wounds cannot be eliminated. Hippocrates can, however, definitively orient the medical skill toward healing and away from elective wounding. He does so by means of speech before others, the *Oath*. Thereby, he founds the medical profession. For a profession is essentially a practice that follows upon, instances, and remains true to what before others one has said one will and will not do. Following Hippocrates' lead, the physician-to-be solemnly commits himself exclusively to promoting the health of the sick. Moreover, he specifies the wounds he will not inflict upon them: in particular, killing, sexual exploitation, and violating confidence. Asclepius' snake forever forswears wounding by taking Hippocrates' *Oath*—to which we now turn.

Chapter 2
HIPPOCRATES' *OATH*

2.1 HIPPOCRATES'?

One could write a book on the appropriateness of the possessive in the title above. This is not such a book. However, the question of the relation between the actual historical physician Hippocrates from the island of Cos who flourished around 434 B.C. and the famous *Oath* merits attention in a work such as this, which articulates the ethic present in the *Oath*. Just as there is a Homeric question, there is also a Hippocratic one. That is, just as scholars debate whether Homer wrote the *Iliad*, so also the well-informed differ as to whether Hippocrates wrote the *Oath*. Indeed, just as historians debate as to whether Homer wrote anything at all, students of the subject differ as to whether Hippocrates wrote anything extant. (As we will see, we can be confident that Hippocrates wrote and that his writings were well known.) The Homeric and the Hippocratic questions importantly differ, however. For all acknowledge the existence of and certain undisputed facts concerning Hippocrates, while some question the very existence of Homer. What do we know about Hippocrates?

A number of texts—two from the works of Plato (Hippocrates' younger contemporary) and one from Aristotle (Plato's student)—serve as trustworthy sources for what we know about the physician from the island of Cos. (Cos itself sits in the Aegean Sea off the southwestern coast of present-day Turkey. Hippocrates presumably inhabited its principal ancient city, Astypalaea, on its southwestern side.) First, let us consider Plato's testimony. The Athenian Plato—who himself lived from 427 to 347 B.C.—informs us about the historical person Hippocrates in dialogues entitled *Protagoras* and *Phaedrus*.

In *Protagoras*, Socrates (469–399 B.C., Hippocrates' contemporary and Plato's teacher) speaks with a young man named Hippocrates (no relation to our Hippocrates—the common-enough name comes from *hippos* "horse" and the suffix *-krates*, from a root meaning "strength" or "power") eager to visit the sophist Protagoras in order to learn—something, he is not entirely sure what—from him for a fee. In light of Hippocrates' ignorance about what he might learn from him, Socrates asks the youth about his desire to study under Protagoras:

[SOCRATES:] Now whom do you think you are going to and what will he make of you? Suppose for instance you had it in mind to go to your namesake Hippocrates of Cos, the doctor [one of the Asclepiads], and pay him a fee on your own behalf, and someone asked you in what capacity you thought of Hippocrates with the intention of paying him, what would you answer?

[HIPPOCRATES:] I should say in his capacity as a doctor.

[SOCRATES:] And what would you hope to become?

[HIPPOCRATES:] A doctor.

[SOCRATES:] And suppose your idea was to go to Polyclitus of Argos or Phidias of Athens and pay them fees for your own benefit, and someone asked you in what capacity you thought of paying this money to them, what would you answer?

[HIPPOCRATES:] I should say, in their capacity as sculptors.

[SOCRATES:] To make you what?

[HIPPOCRATES:] A sculptor, obviously. (Plato 1961, *Protagoras*, 311b3–311c12, 310–11)

From this passage historians (and thoughtful readers) infer that Hippocrates of the island Cos is 1) the most famous and best physician 2) around 434 B.C. who 3) teaches fee-paying students how to doctor, 4) even those unrelated to him. We know (1) that he enjoys the greatest fame as a doctor because Socrates here mentions him in the company of the most famous sculptors to whom a student might go. Moreover, a few lines after this passage, Socrates lets us know that he speaks in "the sort of way that Phidias is called a sculptor and Homer a poet" (311e1–2). That is, illustrative of the best of their kind, as Phidias exemplifies the best sculptor and Homer the best poet. We know (2) because Plato depicts the dialogue as occurring around 434. He does so by referring in the dialogue (which was actually written around 389) to Alcibiades (born in 450) as about sixteen years of age, or at "the most charming age ... the youth with his first beard" (309b). We know (3) that

Hippocrates teaches students how to doctor for a fee from the explicit meaning of the text. We know (4) that Hippocrates teaches unrelated students—a largely unremarked yet important additional conclusion we can draw from this passage—because Socrates proposes that the young man (who coincidentally shares the same name, but apparently not the same family or clan)[1] could readily go to the famous physician and study medicine with him. Indeed, Hippocrates instances the earliest Greek physician known to teach unrelated males for a fee. The teaching of unrelated students merits comment; it will receive greater attention when we consider the *Oath* itself.

Briefly, as Jacques Jouanna (the renowned French medical historian and biographer of Hippocrates) notes, the *Oath* (specifically in light of the contract associated with it, which will receive our attention shortly in 2.2.2) represents a remarkable extension of medical teaching beyond the traditional boundaries whereby (exclusively male) physicians taught only members of the same male lineage (formulaically, "by male descent": Jouanna 1991, 10).[2] In doing so they followed the lead of Asclepius, who taught the healing art to his sons Machaon and Podalirius, both of whom Homer refers to in the *Iliad* as physicians (Homer 1999b, ii, 731–2). Paradigmatically, a physician teaches his son(s) medicine. Jouanna proposes that the extension of medical education beyond the traditional custom of father-teaching-son in part explains why the community of practice associated with the *Oath* survived while others did not, such as that on the island of Rhodes. By enabling a practitioner to teach unrelated males, the *Oath* conferred a number of significant advantages upon those affiliated with it. Consider three benefits realized by one who taught unrelated males along the lines limned by the *Oath's* contractual element.

First, the contract maximized the amount of time during which a practitioner could teach, since, as the practice of medicine was often itinerant, a physician who did have a son whom he could teach had to wait until the youth could accompany him on his travels (as noted in 1.1, literally "epidemiological" from or around—*epi*—one village—*dēmos*—to another) before he could begin to share his art with his offspring. Second, given the contract, a healer lacking sons could still transmit his know-how. This, in turn, conferred some security upon him in his old age, because he could contractually rely upon his former apprentices for aid if he fell into need in a society in which, otherwise, one could depend solely on family. As Plutarch notes in his *Lives* 22.1, the Athenian lawmaker Solon legislated circa 594 B.C.—apparently, to encourage instruction in the crafts—that a son was not obliged to support a father in his senescence if the father had not ensured that his son was taught a livelihood. Third, it assured a physician and his dependent family members that, were death or disability to befall him before he taught the art to a son, his apprentice would (being bound by the contractual element in the *Oath*). Moreover, the agreement conferred these advantages in a milieu in which other traditions of medical practice (such as the above-noted Rhodian) were known to have passed out of existence.[3]

Socrates' remarks in *Protagoras* indicate that the historical Hippocrates shared a distinctive practice with what one finds in the *Oath*—the teaching of the art to unrelated males. More importantly, given that Hippocrates certainly did teach unrelated males, he would have required of them a contract to secure the above-noted benefits for himself and his family. Moreover, in light of the ancient Greeks' affinity for oaths—the historian Judith Fletcher aptly describes them as "the most promise-conscious society on record" (Fletcher 2012, 2)—the tradition to which Hippocrates belonged would have required a solemn vow even of students of male descent. (What I will refer to as the "oath-proper," which contains the ethical commitments to patients, is explicated in 2.2.3). That is, Hippocrates himself would have at one time taken an oath-proper, presumably upon his initiation into medical practice by his father. Thus, it can reasonably be held that Hippocrates wrote a contract for teaching medicine to unrelated males and conjoined the contract with a preexisting oath-proper. The *Oath* has both characteristics; it incorporates a contract for unrelated males and an oath-proper. These salient shared similarities suggest Hippocrates as a plausible author. (Needless to say, in terms of dialect and date—Ionic Greek around the fifth century B.C., discerned in terms of verbal forms and allied evidence—the *Oath* comports with Hippocrates as author.)

To reiterate, from Plato's *Protagoras* we learn that around 434 B.C. Hippocrates of Cos was the best and most famous physician, who, additionally, taught medicine to unrelated male students for a fee. Let us consider the next Platonic treatment of Hippocrates, found in the dialogue *Phaedrus*.

In *Phaedrus* we find out what a student who paid him a fee might have learned from Hippocrates. In the relevant passage in a dialogue ostensibly about erotic love (*eros*) which actually addresses the right use of rhetoric,

Socrates and Phaedrus speak about an analogy between the arts of rhetoric and of medicine in their shared need to "be scientific and not content with mere empirical routine" (Plato 1961, *Phaedrus*, 270b5). At this point we find an allusion to one of the doctrines Hippocrates teaches:

[SOCRATES:] Then do you find it possible to understand the nature of the soul satisfactorily without taking it as a whole?

[PHAEDRUS:] If we are to believe Hippocrates, the Asclepiad, we can't understand even the body without such a procedure.

[SOCRATES:] No, my friend, and he is right. But we must not just rely on Hippocrates; we must examine the assertion and see whether it accords with the truth.

[PHAEDRUS:] Yes.

[SOCRATES:] Then what is it that Hippocrates and the truth have to say on this matter of nature? I suggest that the way to reflect about the nature of anything is as follows: first, to decide whether the object in respect of which we desire to have scientific knowledge, and to be able to impart it to others, is simple or complex, secondly, if it is simple, to enquire what natural capacity it has of acting upon another thing, and through what means; or by what other thing and through what means, it can be acted upon; or, if it is complex, to enumerate its parts and observe in respect of each what we observe in the case of the simple object. [Plato 1961, *Phaedrus*, 270c1–d10]

Here, we discover a number of things about our quarry. First, the text identifies Hippocrates as a member of a clan, the Asclepiad (as he was also described in the *Protagoras*). The Asclepiad are male descendants of

Asclepius (the Greek demigod of medicine), regardless of their occupation. Prior to Hippocrates' extension of medical education to those outside it, doctoring typically entailed being of the Asclepiad clan. Indeed, one often (correctly) translates Asclepiad as "doctor" (as is the case in the previously cited text from *Protagoras*). Second, Hippocrates has a specific written teaching concerning the body's relation to some or *the* (it is not entirely clear) whole. At the very least, that teaching amounts to holding that one must understand the whole in order to proceed methodically and scientifically. Third, Hippocrates writes down and promulgates this doctrine in such a way that it is adequately familiar to Plato's audience for him to employ it in the development of an analogy. Fourth, and finally, Hippocrates acts as an authority to be relied upon to buttress Plato's own account.

Relying on this passage from the *Phaedrus* in their search for Hippocrates' authentic works, historians look at treatises in the Hippocratic corpus (works associated with Hippocrates' school but not necessarily by him, and sometimes assuredly not by him) to see if such a doctrine can be found. Generally, scholars think that a treatise illustrating the doctrine merits attribution to Hippocrates, other things being equal. If other texts can be shown to be by the same author based on other considerations such as style, language, and so on, then they, too, can be associated with Hippocrates. The above represents an important part of the process historians follow in an attempt to establish a work as by Hippocrates.

Unfortunately, as Jouanna notes concerning the tempting text of *Phaedrus*:

> Plato's account brings no clear light to bear on the identification of authentic writings. The only conclusion that emerges from it with certainty is that Hippocrates' method was already famous enough during his lifetime that one of Socrates' interlocutors could refer to it as something well known. (Jouanna 1999, 59)

The *Phaedrus* may not help identify authentic Hippocratic texts. With respect to the authorship of the *Oath*, however, it is not the content of the Hippocratic teaching (whatever that may be) that has significance. Rather, it is the ascription of theoretical medical writings to Hippocrates that has import. For the *Oath* explicitly refers to written teachings (as will be noted in 2.2.2). Thus, the *Phaedrus* sustains the possible identification of Hippocrates with the author of the *Oath*. Let us now turn to our final witness, the student whom Plato is said to have called *nous* (meaning "mind")—Aristotle.

In his *Politics*, Aristotle writes:

> For a state like other things has a certain function to perform, so that it is the state most capable of performing this function that is to be deemed the greatest, just as one would pronounce Hippocrates to be greater, not as a human being, but as a physician, than somebody who surpassed him in bodily size. (Aristotle 1990b, 1326a12–17, 555)

Simply put, Hippocrates is the greatest physician (albeit, apparently, a short man). This is high praise, particularly when one recalls that

Aristotle's father, Nicomachus, was an accomplished physician, serving at the court of Amyntas II, the king of Macedonia. As Jouanna notes, that Aristotle (in a text following the *Phaedrus* by—give or take—four decades) need mention only the physician's name (absent his clan and polis) proves "an unchallenged celebrity" (Jouanna 1999, 7).

Some call forth one further witness to Hippocrates, Aristophanes (448–388 B.C.)—the incomparable comic poet who lampooned Socrates for having his head in the clouds. In Aristophanes' comedy entitled *Thesmophoriazusae* (*Demeter's Festival* or *Festival of the Women*), the tragic poet Euripides coaxes a kinsman to dress up as a woman, attend the women-only festival in honor of Demeter, and prevent the revenge of the women upon him that Euripides fears in light of the misogyny found in his tragedies. Fearing that his disguise will fail and he will be found out (as, of course, does happen, with hilarious effect), Euripides' kinsman seeks an oath from Euripides himself. In the fifth scene, we find the following exchange between the tragic playwright and his unnamed kinsman:

EURIPIDES: You look for all the world like a woman. But when you talk, take good care to give your voice a woman's tone.

KINSMAN: I'll try my best.

EURIPIDES: Come, get yourself to the temple.

KINSMAN: No, by Apollo, not unless you swear to me. . .

EURIPIDES: What?

KINSMAN: . . . that, if anything untoward happen to me, you will leave nothing undone to save me.

EURIPIDES: Very well! I swear it by the Aether, the house of god.

KINSMAN: Why not rather swear it by the housing-flats of Hippocrates?

EURIPIDES: Well then, I swear it by all the gods, both great and small
   (*Thesmophoriazusae*, 266–274).[4]

Here we have an intriguing conjunction of the act of swearing an oath
with someone named Hippocrates. The play dates to 411 B.C. Thus,
if this were a reference to the physician Hippocrates circa 434 B.C.,
it would be clear evidence that he wrote an oath. It would be going
much too quickly, however, to hold that this is such a reference. The
favored explanation refers us to *The Clouds*—one of Aristophanes'
prior plays dating to 423 B.C., in which he ridicules Socrates. There
we find the following reference to a Hippocrates (as previously noted,
a common enough name): "if you shall believe him in this, O youth,
by Bacchus, you will be like the sons of Hippocrates, and they will call
you a booby (Hickie 1853, line 1001)." Which Hippocrates has fool-
ish sons? An (anonymous) early commentator on the text tells us that
Aristophanes here refers to an Athenian Hippocrates who had three,
rude, ignorant sons. Some commentators encountering the reference to
Hippocrates in *Demeter's Festival* of 411 propose that we have the same
Hippocrates. Others suggest that in a play from a dozen years later, it is
probably a different Hippocrates, albeit not our physician. Still others
hold that we do, indeed, here encounter a reference to Hippocrates of
Cos, the author of an oath, and, thus, presumably, the *Oath*. Certainly,
Aristophanes' reference remains a tempting possibility for those seek-
ing to connect Hippocrates of Cos with an oath and, thereby, the *Oath*.

As in the case of temptations more generally, one most likely does best to note the allure while resisting it. In sum, Aristophanes does not serve as an entirely sound witness to Hippocrates as the author of the *Oath*.

So, in light of the testimonies of Hippocrates' younger contemporary Plato and Plato's student Aristotle, what can we make of the historical person Hippocrates of Cos, of the Asclepian clan? From their mentioning of his name, we know that Hippocrates was famous in his own time and even more so shortly thereafter. (Indeed, their writing and speaking about him literally constituted his fame, insofar as to be famous is to be spoken and written about.) Further, the greatest physician, he taught the medical art to unrelated males for a fee; concerning that art, he had written and disseminated a theoretical account.

As my comments suggest, I incline toward thinking that Hippocrates did author the *Oath*, particularly in light of Socrates in *Phaedrus* testifying to Hippocrates' practice of teaching students not related to him for a fee. Extending the medical art in that way would be a momentous departure from traditional practice. Certainly, this novelty required a contract to guarantee that the teacher derived benefit from the unrelated student. Moreover, given ancient Greeks' proclivity for oath-taking—as noted, "the most promise-conscious society on record" (Fletcher 2012, 2)—we can be confident that medical students swore an oath, regardless of descent. Such considerations suggest a greater than even likelihood that Hippocrates did author the *Oath*.[5]

A reader reasonably asks: what difference does it make? Is the question not largely academic? While bookish, the question has more than scholarly import. For, if the *Oath* is Hippocratic, then medical practice in its very origins jointly emphasizes technical and ethical norms: medical expertise serving health exclusively. Regardless of its actual author, the *Oath* exemplifies perennial profound insights into medical practice vis-à-vis the human condition. To it, I now turn.

2.2 *OATH*: GODS, GODDESSES, CONTRACT, AND OATH-PROPER

Horkos, the Greek word for "oath," is related to *herkos* "fence, that which encloses." Of course, an oath binds the juror (oath-taker) to act only within a defined field of activity. As one scholar notes: "*Horkos* is also a cognate of *exorkismos* (exorcism), which puts evil things and persons 'outside the fence'" (Plescia 1970, 2). Putting certain things outside the fence renders the enclosed space fit for the activity on account of which it has been reserved. Just as the bounds of a soccer pitch (or any field of play) allow the game to take place, an oath establishes boundaries for important activities. *Horkos* can also refer to either that by which one swears (e.g., the heavens) or one who witnesses such swearing (a god). By extension, it comes to mean the actual oath one swears.

Taking the *Oath* as a whole, first, we meet the relevant gods by whom one swears; second, we encounter details that concern the contract (in Greek *sungraphē*; literally, something written [*graphē*] with [*syn*] another, a written agreement); third, and finally, we find specifics regarding what I refer to as the oath-proper. As we will see, the contract principally concerns the student's obligations to his teacher. The oath-proper bears on the juror's obligations to the sick. Before explicating these parts, I wish briefly to consider general features of oath-taking as practiced by the Greeks.

The Greek practice of swearing an oath had three elements: those (or that) by whom (or which) one swears, that to which one swears, and the punishment that will result if one swears falsely. Given the solemnity of oath-taking, people typically swore by the highest beings, the gods and goddesses. When it comes to that to which one swears, we find two kinds of oaths, testimonial and promissory.

A testimonial oath resembles the commonly encountered judicial practice of swearing in witnesses, for example, on a bible, to tell the "truth, the whole truth, and nothing but the truth." A promissory oath concerns the future performance of that to which one swears. Exclusively addressing the juror's future conduct, the *Oath* is promissory. While it is in this respect similar to contemporary wedding vows—"to have and to hold, from this day forward, for better, for worse, for richer, for poorer, in sickness and in health, until death do us part"—one caveat must be issued. While the Greek promissory oath (by definition) includes a promise to do (or avoid) certain acts, it also characteristically incorporates the calling down of a penalty by the juror upon himself if he does not fulfill the promise. Thus, we find oaths (typically) explicitly including the oath-takers wishing harm upon themselves were they to violate the oath, a conditional self-cursing. In this respect, the promissory oath partially resembles sworn testimony, which usually includes some explicit recognition that the testifier swears "under penalty of perjury." However, even this recognition of the penalty of perjury does not capture the contingent self-curse of the Greek promissory oath, for the Greek promissory oath has the juror positively request punishment for violating it. It would be akin to testifying in court and saying, "May I suffer conviction for perjury if my testimony is false." As a student of Greek oaths notes, the gravity of the self-curse partially indicates the sacredness of the oath (Plescia 1970, 12). Thus, as we shall see when we consider the grievousness of the self-curse found therein, the *Oath* has a high degree of solemnity. With these preliminaries in place, let us consider the witnesses called forth by the juror.

2.2.1 *Gods and Goddesses*

Here begins the *Oath* (translated literally and, as much as possible, following the Greek word-order; the entire *Oath* and Greek text with this literal translation can be found in the appendix):

> I swear by Apollo physician and Asclepius and Hygeia and Panacea and by both all the gods and all [the goddesses], making [them my] witnesses, to fulfill according to my ability and judgement this oath and this contract;

In the first person, the oath-taker swears (using the form *omnumi*, in keeping with fifth-century oaths, and not *omnuo*, more common in the fourth century, as remarked by Fletcher 2012, 6)—in the following order—by Apollo healer (or physician), Asclepius, Hygeia, Panacea, and (as is customary) all the gods and (as is not customary) goddesses.[6] Having sworn by them, he makes them his witnesses that he will fulfill according to his ability and judgement the following oath and contract. Who are the named gods and goddesses? Let us consider them in their order of precedence. Before doing so, we note an omnipresent, although not specifically named god, Zeus Horkios, the god of oaths. For "all oaths are under the stewardship of Zeus *Horkios*" (Fletcher 2012, 5).

First, we encounter Apollo, healer (or physician). As noted in 1.3, the *Oath* specifies Apollo in this particular role because he plays numerous parts, including some opposed to medicine, such as the god of plague and disease. Myth proposes that Apollo—"most Greek of all gods"—fathered Asclepius by Coronis.[7] Upon learning from a crow that Coronis had been unfaithful to him, Apollo had her killed, turned the crow black, and took away its ability to sing. While Coronis' corpse burned on the funeral pyre, Apollo removed Asclepius from her womb (thus, rather than the Caesarian we might speak of the Asclepian section). Apollo had the mythical centaur Chiron instruct Asclepius in the medical arts. The name Chiron probably comes from the Greek *cheir*, meaning "hand." By definition, Chiron is a *cheirourgos*, one who works (*ergon* "work, action") with his hands; medically, a surgeon. Indeed, "surgeon" is an Anglicization of the Greek; Shakespeare employs "chirurgeonly" for "surgeonly" (*The Tempest* 2.1.141). As some historians note, Chiron (intriguingly, given his association with the medical art) also first instructed men in the swearing of oaths (Fletcher 2012, 1). (In chapter 4, I argue on behalf of a close connection between medicine and oath-taking, perhaps intimated by Chiron's dual roles.) Let us now consider our second witness, Apollo's son Asclepius.

In the *Iliad*, Homer (twice) refers to the mortal Asclepius as the "excellent physician (199b, iv, 194; xi, 518)." In both instances, Homer uses *amumonos*, literally meaning "without blame"; the word (never used of gods) has an honorific title-like character, like our "the honorable." As noted previously, in keeping with the family practice the Homeric Asclepius has two physician-sons, Machaon and Podalirius (*Iliad*, ii, 732), whom he would have himself educated in the medical art per the custom of his day (from which his most famous descendant would depart). By the time of Pindar's *Odes* (approximately three centuries after the *Iliad*), the mortal hero will have been divinized into the Greek demigod by whom our oath-taker swears. Asclepius is the demigod of health, founder of the Asclepiad clan, supplicated in numerous Asclepieia (temples devoted to his cult, the singular being Asclepieion). The principal temple was on the Peloponnesian peninsula in Epidauros. Now a UNESCO world-heritage site, it dates to the seventh century B.C. In 420 B.C., Asclepius' cult came to Athens, where his temple rose on the south slope of the Acropolis, on land "highly desirable, restricted, and regulated" (Wickkiser 2008, 76). Interestingly, part of the increase in the importance of Asclepius' cult (as indicated by the prominence given to the Athenian Asclepieion) can be attributed to the unwillingness of trained physicians to treat those whom they regarded as incurable. As one historian of devotion to Asclepius explains:

> in the late fifth century and fourth century, as Hippocratic treatises continued to emphasize the limits of medical practice, Asklepios' cult rapidly became one of the most popular

healing cults in all of antiquity, spreading to numerous places both within and outside of Greece. (Wickkiser 2008, 41)

Anyone swearing to Asclepius could do so in good faith vis-à-vis the god, for the physician-in-training would learn to distinguish the medically curable from the incurable. With respect to the latter, he might piously suggest recourse to the god (Wickkiser 2008, 33). Hence the rise of Asclepius' cult coincides with that of competent medical practitioners. (One ritual a supplicant might undergo would be to sleep in the Asclepieion after receiving a soporific drink. If his prayers were answered, the sleeping petitioner would dream of the god revealing the cure.)

Before moving on to consider the other properly named gods, one notes that the father and son pairing of Apollo-healer and Asclepius encountered at the very beginning of the *Oath* emphasizes the father-educating-son medical tradition from which the *Oath* both arises and (in imparting medical education to unrelated males) departs. Let us now consider Asclepius' children by and before whom the juror swears.

Hygeia (her name, also spelled Hygieia, means "health," and from it we derive the word "hygiene") is a goddess, the daughter of Asclepius and Epione (whose name means "soothing").[8] As her own name indicates, Hygeia personifies health itself. After Hygeia, we encounter her sister, the goddess Panacea. Her name derives from the Greek *pan*, meaning "all," and *akos* meaning "cure" or "remedy," from which we derive "panacea," a cure-all. Thus, Panacea would be the ancillary goddess aiding the physician especially in the use of healing substances such as salves, compresses, and so on. While her name has come narrowly to refer to what we would conceive of as drugs, as understood by the oath-taker she would be the goddess, broadly, of any physical means used to cure. When we turn to the oath-proper, we will see the juror swear to benefit the sick by the use of regimens (*diaitēma*), etymologically "what has been divided" (e.g., portions of food, medicaments, extended to include, broadly, treatments). Panacea would be the goddess of physical materials employed in treatment of the sick. So, for example, in Aristophanes' comedic play entitled *Plutus* (*Wealth*, which remains the most informative source for the incubation, or laying in, that occurred at an Asclepieion), Panacea assists Asclepius by covering the slumbering Plutus' head and face with a purple cloth (*Plutus*, line 731, Aristophanes 2002, 530–1).

Finally—for good measure, as it were—the oath-taker swears "by all the gods and goddesses." "By all the gods" amounts to something of a standard line ending the list of the divines by whom the oath-taker swears. By contrast, as noted, oaths rarely include "and [all the] goddesses." Having duly treated of the gods and goddesses, let us now consider the specifics of the contract.

2.2.2 Contract

The *Oath* includes a *sungraphē*, a contract. The written agreement enables the practitioner to teach an unrelated male student while insuring that by doing so the physician will realize benefits comparable to those realized by teaching a son. To appreciate the significance of this aspect of the contract, recall the law (noted in 2.1) that Solon promulgated requiring that an Athenian son support his elderly needy father, if that father had secured instruction in an occupation for the son. The contract enables a physician (regardless of how he stands in terms of sons) to secure his old age. In a society in which the family serves as the sole source of material support for the needy, the physician who teaches an unrelated male needs to insure that the unrelated student will support him and his family (if necessary) as a son would (and in some cases due to laws such as Solon's, must). The contract insures the fulfillment of this vital function. By the terms of the contract, the former student must support the teacher just as a son must support a needy elderly father who had secured a livelihood for him. Moreover, as noted, if the teacher does have sons it provides some assurance that were he to die (or become disabled) before teaching them, they would receive instruction in the art and the livelihood such instruction confers. Let us look at the contractual elements more closely.

Immediately after calling to witness "all the gods and goddesses," the juror articulates the contractual terms concerning his teacher:

> to regard indeed my teacher in this art as equal to my parents, and of my livelihood to share [with him], and [to him] needing necessities to make [him] a share [of mine], and his male offspring to esteem as equal to [my] brothers, and to teach [them] this art, if they want to learn [it], without fee and contract, of rule and lecture and all remaining teaching I will make a share with my sons and those of my teacher, and with students contracted and oathed to the physician's law, but to not one other.

If we look simply at the contractual elements of the *Oath*, we find the following sequence of obligations. First, when necessary, to meet the needs of "him who taught me this art." As the contract stipulates, he is to treat his teacher as if he were a parent. Second, concerning the teacher's sons, the one contracted will teach those willing to learn the art, without fee or contract. The student will treat the teacher's sons as if they were his own. By contrast, not being the teacher's son, the student both pays tuition and incurs contractual obligations. Third, in terms of content, the student will teach by means of "[written] rule and lecture and all remaining teaching." (The word translated here as "rule" (*parangeliēs*) suggests a contrast to that translated as "lecture" (*akroēsios*), meaning "what one listens to," so that we are to understand it to refer to what is written down in contrast to what is spoken. Hence the *Oath* belongs to a tradition having written medical teachings.) Fourth, and finally, by these means he will teach his own sons, those of his teacher (as heretofore pledged), and students (such as himself) "contracted and oathed to the physician's custom" (*nomō iētrikō—nomos* means "custom," "usage," or "law;" *iētrikos* means "iatric," "having to do with a physician," or "medical") but "to not one other."

As noted, the contract binds the unrelated student as if he were a son. Notably, sons of the teacher need not sign the contract nor pay him if the unrelated physician becomes their teacher. Also meriting remark, someone outside the clan of Asclepiads who becomes a physician can teach his own sons—of course, free of contract and fee. The *Oath* (incorporating the contract) explicitly refers to three categories of students: the juror's sons, the teacher's sons, and students such as the juror "contracted and oathed to the physician's (or medical) custom (or law)."

With respect to the oath to the law of medicine—the oath-proper—a number of questions arise. Had the teacher himself (not contracted) previously sworn the oath-proper or its equivalent? Although the student-sons of physicians need not sign the contract nor pay a fee, would they be required to swear to the medical law? (Of course, the juror himself does.)

In answering these questions, recall that the medical tradition prior to the *Oath* restricts instruction to the male lineage. The physician's custom (referred to as established) cannot be this new practice of contracting unrelated males. Rather, the medical custom or law predates the *Oath* fashioned for the teaching of unrelated males and comprised of both the contract and oath-proper. This points to a medical law standing as something preexisting and separate from the contract. Given this passage and the Greeks noted affinity for oaths, it is safe to assume that in the tradition to which the *Oath* belongs, prior to its introduction, practitioners swore to uphold the medical *nomos*. Thus, the teacher, his sons, and those of the juror (while not bound by contract, nor required to pay tuition) are oathed to the medical custom (*nomō iētrikō*). Certainly, we encounter that normative custom (or its descendant) in the oath-proper, which presents the physician's obligations to the sick (of which we will treat extensively in 2.2.3).

To consider the implications of the contract and oath-proper in terms of actual Hippocratic doctors, contrast Hippocrates' student and most renowned son, Thessalus, and his (more famous) student and son-in-law, Polybus (the author of *Nature of Man*, a work in the Hippocratic corpus which presents the famous theory of the four humors: phlegm, blood, black bile, and yellow bile). Thessalus would have oathed himself to the custom of medicine (either by the oath-proper or its equivalent) but would not have taken the *Oath* (including the contract), while Polybus would have taken the *Oath*, inclusive of the contract and oath-proper. Their sons would not have differed in this respect, for they would promise to follow the medical custom (oath-proper) while being instructed without fee or contract—as had their famous grandfather. The sons of Thessalus and Polybus would have differed, however, in another way meriting (brief) remark.

In addition to the Hippocratic *Oath* we find another oath associated with (but not inaugurated by) Hippocrates. This oath concerns certain religious privileges at Delphi enjoyed by the aforementioned Asclepiads. Presumably due to Hippocrates' radical step and the associated increasing numbers of non-Asclepiad physicians who might (falsely) claim full membership in the clan, the Asclepiads of Cos and of Cnidus required an oath of those claiming the religious privileges while at Delphi. The juror swore that he was indeed an Asclepiad by male descent (Jouanna 1999, 33–5). Hence, Thessalus and any of his sons could, while Polybus and his sons could not, honestly take this oath if they went to Delphi (as Hippocrates himself apparently did).

To reiterate, we can be confident that practitioners in the medical tradition out of which the *Oath* arises practiced in accordance with the mentioned custom. We can be confident of this because the *Oath* is the novel means by which practitioners incorporate new members into their heretofore entirely familial practice. Accordingly, just as the contract attempts to render the unrelated student (e.g., Polybus) equivalent to a son (e.g., Thessalus), so also the oath-proper serves to insure that the new member abides by the norms governing practitioners in relation to those with whom they have always had a relationship—namely, the sick. Thus, one finds the innovation of the *Oath* not so much in its famous moral content articulating the physician's obligations to the sick (for those commitments certainly predate the *Oath*), but rather in the extension by contract of medical education beyond kinship. As Jouanna remarks, "Paradoxically, the welcoming of foreign students into the family could serve to perpetuate the familial tradition" (1999, 48). Indeed, Hippocrates' son-in-law Polybus perfectly illustrates the truth of this paradox, since history indicates that he surpassed his brother-in-law Thessalus (and Draco, Hippocrates' other son) in preserving and advancing medicine. Hippocrates wisely departed from tradition and thereby sustained and furthered medicine's practice and the medical law, custom, or ethic.

Yet why extend instruction beyond the traditional family boundaries? Both the lack of demand for instruction among physicians' sons and its presence among the more general population explain this extension. As noted, if one limits instruction to male descent, one thereby significantly reduces the opportunity to pass on knowledge of medical practice. Some physicians will simply not have the requisite sons. Moreover, among the sons of physicians, some will not be fit due to age or inability, others will not want to practice the art, and so on.

In short, the vagaries of sustaining any familial tradition will naturally beset that of the Asclepiads. As for the presence of demand among unrelated males, as the text of the *Phaedrus* indicates, others not in the family will want to learn the art and may request instruction. Certainly, Solon's (noted) law encouraging fathers to instruct their sons in arts conferring a livelihood conduces to increased demand for medical education among non-doctoring families.

Jouanna notes such causes for extending medical education beyond unrelated males:

> According to a *Commentary on the Oath* attributed to Galen, Hippocrates decided to make instruction available to strangers owing to an insufficient number of family members willing to carry on the medical tradition of Cos, and drafted the *Oath* to this effect. This explanation deserves to be taken seriously. The Asclepiads of Cos were well aware of their relatives on the neighboring island of Rhodes, where the medical tradition had died out. . . . It is also possible that the reputation of the physicians trained in the family of the Asclepiads brought about this enlargement; in any case, the renown of Hippocrates favored it, if it did not actually cause it to occur. (1999, 47–8)

Regardless of its causes, we can be confident (given the Greeks' noted oath-taking proclivity) that upon the revolutionary opening up of the practice to those outside the family, the new associate would vow to abide by the tradition's norms. Accordingly, having treated of the contract, we now turn to the aforementioned oath-proper, which embodies the medical custom.

2.2.3.1 Oath-Proper: Regimens, Harm, and Injustice

Here follows the beginning of the oath-proper:

> Regimens [*diaitēmasî*] I will use for the benefit of the sick [*kamnontōn*] according to my ability and judgment, but [what is used] for harm [*dēlēsei*] and injustice [*adikiēi*] I will keep away from [the sick].

Here we first encounter the beneficiaries of the oath-proper, the sick. As noted, the contract with which the *Oath* begins principally concerns itself with the welfare of the teacher (and, by extension, his sons). The teacher now leaves the stage, no longer to be mentioned. From this point, the sick alone matter. To refer to the sick, the oath-proper uses the Greek *kamnontōn* (here and subsequently when speaking of going into houses, again using the same phrase "for the benefit of the sick"). This word is a form of the verb *kamnō*, meaning "to work," "to be weary," or "to be sick." The participial form found in the oath-proper can in other contexts also refer to those who have entirely completed their work: the dead. By extension, it refers to those laboring, as it were, under an illness: the sick. (Of course, we typically speak of those for whom physicians care as patients, from the Latin verb *patior*, to suffer or undergo. Hence the Greek and Latin words both suggest that the ill bear sickness.)

For the benefit of the sick, the juror will use regimens (*diaitēmata*). As noted in 2.2.1 in our discussion of the goddess Panacea, this word originally means "what has been divided." It comes to mean, variously, what is cut up and divided, portions of food, dietary measures, medicaments, physical treatments, and, by extension, therapies more generally. While not limited to physical therapeutic items, it does focus on concrete materials (as we shall see in the specific exclusion of giving a deadly drug or a destructive pessary).

Next, we come upon the phrase "according to my ability and judgment," now exercised in the use of therapies for the benefit of the sick. The phrase recalls the aforementioned limitations that Hippocratically trained medical practitioners appear to have readily acknowledged. It strikes a reader as an honest, humble self-assessment as the one who vows begins his apprenticeship. (As noted, the acknowledgment of medicine's limits, conjoined with a willingness to refer those not Hippocratically curable to the care of Asclepius, benefits the god's cult.)

Having promised that he will act for the benefit of the sick, the oath-taker correspondingly pledges not to use harm and injustice in his dealings with the sick. Rather, he will keep harm and injustice away from the sick. The Greek word here translated as "harm" (*dēlēsei*) (our word "deleterious" derives from the same Greek root) refers to damage, mischief, ruin, or bane. It extends to both inadvertent and intentional harming. As it refers to accidental harming, it comports with the aforementioned "at least do no harm" principle (briefly discussed in 1.2). *Adikiē* refers to injustice, deliberate wrongdoing. It would not encompass doing something that adventitiously hurts another. Accordingly, we should understand the *Oath* to commit the taker of it to preserving patients from both injury (where intent is understood to be absent) and injustice (where intent is present). This generic commitment precedes a specific listing of the more salient hurts and wrongs—especially as they are physically instanced—from which the vow-taker will safeguard the sick, prominently among which we find the two most famous, namely the giving or suggesting of a deadly drug and the giving of an abortive.

2.2.3.2 Oath-Proper: The Rejection of Killing

First, let us consider a literal translation of the relevant passage:

> I will neither give a deadly drug to anyone, though having been asked,
> nor will I lead the way to such counsel;
> and, similarly, to a woman a destructive pessary I will not give.
> But purely and piously I will watch over my life and my art.

This passage clearly parallels the one mentioning "regimens" or material therapies employed for the benefit of the sick. As a foil to beneficial physical therapies, we here find obnoxious materials: a deadly drug and a destructive pessary. These instance harmful and unjust physical media not to be used upon, but, rather, to be warded off from the sick. The juror forswears both. These pledges not to give a deadly drug and not to give a destructive (abortive) pessary cannot be understood absent the juror's concluding reference to purely and piously guarding his life and art. Let us begin there.

The Greek word for "purely" (*hagnōs*), coming as it does after reference to not giving a deadly drug and not giving a life-destroying abortive, indicates that the *Oath* here addresses purity from blood-guilt. That is, the oath-taker forswears killing and thus will be pure before all the gods and goddesses in this respect (and not, for example, sexually chaste, another connotation *hagnōs* can have in other contexts, e.g., when said of a maiden). This sense of being free from blood on one's hands before the gods becomes even more pronounced when one considers the complementing word for that here translated as "piously," *hosiōs*. The adjective *hosios* contrasts with *dikaios*, whose root we have already encountered in the phrase, "[what is used] for harm and injustice (*adikiē*) I will keep away from [the sick]." *Dikaios* refers to human justice; *hosios* refers to righteousness before and with the gods. Indeed, one of the most famous Platonic dialogues (*Euthyphro*) features a conversation exclusively about what is *hosios* between Socrates and a young, religiously minded Euthyphro (his name means "orthodox" or "right-minded," from *euthys* "right" or "straight" and *phrēn* "heart; mind; wits").

Briefly, to Socrates' (and Euthyphro's entire family's) dismay, Euthyphro prosecutes his own father for the death of a hired worker who himself while drunk had killed one of the family's slaves. While waiting for word from the religious authority on what to do with the killer, Euthyphro's father binds and leaves him unprovided for in a ditch, where he dies of hunger and cold. Euthyphro prosecutes his father lest he himself suffer blood guilt (*miasma*). Claiming to know what is *hosios* (a knowledge Socrates regards as belonging to one far advanced in wisdom), Euthyphro takes his father to court for the murderous worker's death. Plato portrays Euthyphro as an ignorant, unjustifiably theologically opinionated, reckless individual who serves as a foil to

Socrates. By contrast, Socrates repeatedly examines what he thinks he knows and does not know, treads cautiously concerning divine matters, and cares for others' welfare (especially that of his fellow Athenians).[9] Of course, Euthyphro represents an unreasonable obsession with an otherwise appropriate concern to avoid blood on one's hands. For our purposes, the dialogue nicely illustrates the conventionally perceived connection between righteousness before the gods (*hosios*) with freedom from blood-guilt. Accordingly, the *Oath* features a religious sensibility that forswears killing (including inchoate human life).

With freedom from blood-guilt before the gods in mind, the apprentice-physician pledges not to give a deadly drug to anyone if asked for it, nor to suggest such a course of action. There is, of course, much to discuss here. Moreover, given how fraught with moral import this passage is, controversy attends the conversation. Least controversially, the text itself supports a number of inferences. First, practitioners in the tradition to which the *Oath* belongs had lethal drugs at their disposal. Second, others knew this and requested such drugs. Third, given the proximity to the preceding promise to keep what is harmful and unjust away from the sick, those belonging to and joining this practice regard giving such drugs as harmful and unjust. Moreover, given the noted subsequent passage concerning purity and piety as they bear on blood-guilt, the juror regards complicity in the giving of a deadly drug as blood-guilt-ridden and impious. Further salient questions require more extensive treatment.

First, to whom will the physician not give a deadly drug? Who asks for the lethal substance? Second, and following on our answer to the first question, what counsel or advice (the Greek word is *boulē*, meaning "counsel," "advice," or "plan") will the physician not give? Before answering these questions, I note that the oath-taker (emphatically) will not give a deadly drug to anyone; literally "to not one." Thus, in focusing our interpretation we do not thereby suggest that the physician is somehow open to giving deadly drugs otherwise. Nonetheless, the one promising has something specific in mind here, as the rejection of suggesting "such advice" indicates.

Who, precisely, requests a deadly drug? We have a number of plausible candidates: first, a patient requesting a deadly drug for himself; second, a third party requesting a deadly drug for a patient; third, a person other than a patient requesting a deadly drug for himself; and, fourth and finally, a person (patient or otherwise) requesting a deadly drug in order to kill a person other than a patient. The basic division between the options is that between the request concerning the killing of a patient (either the patient requesting or a third party requesting) and the request not concerning the killing of a patient. Given that the oath-proper here speaks of a doctor and a request for a deadly drug, one reasonably, straightforwardly, and intuitively interprets this as bearing on the killing of a patient. Yet some suggest that the *Oath* here does not address a request concerning the killing of a patient. Rather, they see it as a request to poison someone other than a patient; namely, to murder (or assassinate) one of the general public.[10]

On the face of things implausible, this proposal has the added odd result of the physician vowing not to suggest such killing. Yet, to whom would he not suggest this? Presumably to some third party interested in murder. If this account were correct, it would mean that physicians promised not to suggest the murder of people outside their therapeutic enterprise to people outside their therapeutic enterprise. In addition to requiring such (darkly humorous) officiousness of the physician—officious as the rejection of an act so far removed from the practice of medicine—this seems an unnecessary interpretive reach, for a patient at times desires death and asks this of the physician. Similarly, the family at times thinks a patient's death desirable and asks this of the physician. Thus, we need not stray so far afield to interpret the swearing not to give a deadly drug or counseling the same as referring to the killing of a patient.

Moreover, and most importantly, the Greek text itself calls for this interpretation. In what immediately precedes this passage, the juror swears to use regimens for the benefit of the sick and to keep what is harmful and unjust away from them. Again, the oath-proper reads:

> Regimens [*diaitēmasi*] I will use for the benefit of the sick [*kamnontōn*] according to my ability and judgment, but [what is used] for harm [*dēlēsei*] and injustice [*adikiēi*] I will keep away from [the sick].

In Greek, the words for "regimens," "harm," and "injustice" are in the dative case. (The cases reflect a word's function in a sentence.)[11] In classical Greek, to indicate a thing's instrumental role the dative case is used. In this context, the dative case points to the means or instrument used to achieve a purpose or (in the instance of rejected means) not used. The first clause clearly means that the juror will use regimens for the purpose of benefiting the sick. The second clause has a parallel construction, addressing what the juror will not use concerning the sick. That is, he will not use means ordered toward harm and injustice in his dealings with the sick; rather, he will keep these away from the sick.

Immediately subsequent to this general commitment, and referencing specific materials implicated in harm and injustice to the sick (as a foil to the aforementioned beneficial physical regimens), the oath-taker disavows the use of a specific noxious physical item, namely a deadly drug given to a patient upon request (either by the sick individual or by another). Nor will he counsel that deadly drugs be taken by a patient. Simply put, the Greek text clearly indicates that the juror forswears giving a deadly drug to a patient or advising that the patient take a lethal drug.

The next word (*homoiōs*, meaning "similarly" or "likewise") links the disavowal of giving or suggesting the taking of a deadly drug with the passage concerning a destructive (*pthorion*) pessary (the adjective is related to the verb *phtheirō*, meaning "to destroy"). Thus, the pessary or vaginal plug at issue is abortive. Of course, just as the rejection of the use of deadly drugs implies knowledge concerning such drugs, so also the rejection of a destructive pessary implies such knowledge. The juror swears not to give an abortive pessary to a woman. Some commentators interpret the inclusion of "to a woman" as indicating that the oath-taker restrictively forswears only giving such pessaries to women, leaving open the possibility of giving them to others so that they might be used on women. Others suggest that the rejection is only of destructive pessaries and not of other abortive means. Let us consider these two proposals.

Interpreting "to a woman" restrictively falls short by neglecting the intimate association of this passage with that rejecting deadly drugs and the overarching concern to avoid blood-guilt or being implicated in killing. Moreover, it does not give adequate emphasis to the rejection of the pessary insofar as it is destructive, or abortive. This also highlights the deficiency of those interpretations that would limit the rejection to pessaries while accepting other means, for the oath-proper clearly rejects the relevant pessaries *as destructive*.

"To a woman" here serves to specify the act that is being rejected, namely the destruction of nascent life found, necessarily, within a pregnant woman. The juror avoids being implicated in the taking of inchoate human life and therefore forswears the giving of a destructive pessary to a woman. Wanting to be free of blood before the gods, he promises not to use his art to kill either mature or inchoate human life.

To reiterate, by the oath-proper the juror clearly, categorically, and conclusively rejects killing.

2.2.3.3 Oath-Proper: Cutting

The next passage seems out of place, an odd juxtaposition between the avoidance of blood-guilt and the following two passages addressing the entering of the homes of the sick. It reads as follows:

> I will not cut, indeed [*mēn*], not even on those suffering from stone, but I will give way to practicing men in this doing.

This passage is fraught with difficulties. It flummoxes commentators. By it the juror rejects recourse to surgery. The verb is *temnō*, meaning "to cut." Yet cutting is a well-accepted practice in ancient Greek medicine. Recall, for example, that Chiron, the centaur who taught Asclepius the art of medicine, has a name suggesting "hand," intimately related to the ancient Greek word *cheirourgous*, which literally means "one who works with his hands"—medically, a surgeon. To invoke Asclepius, Chiron's most famous student, while forswearing surgery sounds discordant. Heroic attempts to incorporate this text into the *Oath* itself and into the practice of ancient Greek medicine more generally lead interpreters to make various suggestions. Consider four representative attempts and their respective difficulties. First, that this commitment covers the student only while he is a student—an entirely ad hoc proposal, given the once-and-for-all character of the other commitments. Second, that the text refers to (medically contraindicated) castration. But why acquiesce to the others mentioned who would perform this? Third, that the text refers only to cutting for those suffering from stones—a hopeful solution, but one that neglects the literal text that rejects cutting, *sans phrase*, while singling out "indeed, not even" those suffering from stones. Fourth, and finally, that unrelated males would not cut, while the Asclepiads by male descent would retain the surgical franchise. Yet who would teach their sons without fee or contract were they unable to do so? In short, as the diverse interpretations indicate, this text does not sit well either with the *Oath* itself or with what we know of the ancient Greek medical context out of which it certainly originates. Moreover, the addition of *mēn* (here acting as an intensifier) has an insistent character meaning "honestly," "truly," or "really." Given the deficiencies of the other alternatives, the most plausible position concerning this passage is that it is a late interpolation. A reader of the *Oath* senses the lack of flow and abruptness at this point. This passage remains ectopic; it is not in keeping either with the *Oath* itself or with the tradition to which the *Oath* certainly belongs (regardless of that tradition's relationship to the historical Hippocrates). Having noted its eccentricity, allow me to put further consideration of this passage aside. Indeed, truly, really (if I may so speak of it), it seems not to belong to the *Oath*.

2.2.3.4 Oath-Proper: Entering Houses Free of Injustice (Sexual Acts)

The next passage reads as follows:

> Into as many houses as I enter, I will go into in order to benefit the sick, being free from all voluntary injustice and corruption, especially sexual acts with the bodies of females and of males, of free and of slaves.

As noted, medical practice often involved going from one village to another and typically entailed going into the houses of the sick. House calls were the norm, not the anomaly they have become. The Ancient Greek household characteristically consisted of an extended family. At the center of the extended family were the husband and wife with their unmarried daughters and sons. Farther out from this center were their married sons with their own wives and children, the husband's surviving parents, and, finally, slaves (if any). To give some sense of the import of entering the house, daily prayers were characteristically offered to

Zeus Ktesios (protector of wealth), Zeus Herkeios (protector of the house-boundary), and Apollo Agyieus (protector of the entrance to the house).[12] Thus, for a non-family member to enter a Greek household was in itself a significant act fraught with concerns of threats posed to the household's possessions, occupants, and (as we will shortly see) reputation. In keeping with Greek religion and culture, the juror makes specific promises concerning the salient act of going into the house.

This passage again includes the phrase "benefit of the sick," empha-sizing that entering the household occurs for the good of the sick. Immediately thereafter, the juror swears to remain free of all voluntary injustice (*adikia*) and corruption (*pthoria*). This echoes the preceding promise not to use means ordered toward harm [*dēlēsei*] and injustice [*adikiēi*] when dealing with the sick. Here, the emphasis upon the volun-tary highlights the absence of all malice, scheming, or ulterior purpose. Whoever enters the household as a physician does so entirely without guile, absolutely avoiding injustice and deliberate harm. Thus, the juror disavows moral corruption, or entering the household for some nefari-ous purpose, under the guise of doing so in order to care for the sick.

Further along, the oath-proper specifies injustice and corruption of a venereal nature—or, to provide a more literal translation of the Greek, aphrodisiacal character, Aphrodite being the Greek (and Venus the Roman) goddess of erotic love. Most literally, the juror here swears to avoid "sexual acts upon female and male bodies (*sōmatōn*)." Many translate this as "female and male persons." The Greek has a concrete-ness that the abstract noun (of Latin origin) "persons" does not entirely capture. "Bodies" understandably can strike us as odd, accustomed as we are to the less tangible "persons." (This illustrates the concreteness of Greek in contrast to the abstractness of Latin and of Latin-based English derivatives.) Whatever the case concerning how one translates the relevant term, the juror emphatically abjures all sexual relations with females or males, free or slave in the household.

2.2.3.5 Oath-Proper: Entering Houses and Not Gossiping

The next passage naturally belongs with the preceding that begins with "into as many houses as I may enter." It reads:

> About whatever in therapy I see or hear, or also outside of ther-
> apy concerning the life of men, that ought never to be spoken
> out, I will be silent, holding such things not to be spoken.

The above chiefly concerns the juror's continued promises bearing on his conduct concerning the household's occupants. Of course, this does not mean that the physician will gossip about patients not seen in house-holds. Rather, it reflects the concern over the integrity of the household and its members. The *Oath* commits the practitioner to strict silence with great specificity, concerning what he sees and hears, in exercising caregiving or outside of caregiving. The Greek uses *therapeia* meaning service or care, more specifically, as we continue to use it, medical care, therapy. Thus, we here see the strenuousness of the *Oath*. Regardless of how one came upon the matter that ought not to be spoken of abroad, having been allowed into the household for the benefit of the sick, the physician shall not speak out about the family's private life. The Greek word for speak out is the apt verb *eklaleō*, from *ek-* meaning "out" and the (apparently onomatopoeic) verb *laleō*, meaning "to blurt out," "to chatter." In short, the physician swears to be discrete, worthy of confidence, admissible (without subsequent jeopardy or public embarrassment) into the privacy of one's home and familial life. The physician deems such matters *arrēta*, from a prefix meaning "not" and *rhētos*, meaning "may be spoken." Thus, the physician regards these matters as what ought not to be spoken; to do so is shameful. Of course, the *Oath*-taker does not avoid all speech about these matters, but rather chattering about them abroad, outside the household. Presumably, some of these matters are the very ones on account of which he entered the house in the first place. He will certainly speak of them to some in the household. These matters have the character of being sacred, shared secrets to be discussed among the physician and members of the household. They bear on the family's good reputation, something jealously guarded by most peoples, but especially by the Greeks, for whom what others say about one (one's *doxa*) has great significance. Shortly, we will encounter the aspiration of the juror for good reputation (*doxa*), even fame. Part of his good reputation will depend upon his not harming the good *doxa* concerning anyone else, especially insofar as, given his privilege of entry into households, he may have unique opportunities to harm an individual's or family's reputation by gossip.

2.2.4 The Oath Concludes: Blessing and Self-curse

Finally, we conclude the *Oath* (and the oath-proper) with the (noted) requisite self-curse, one of the distinct features of an oath in Ancient

Greece. We also find (as we at times do elsewhere) a self-blessing. The text reads as follows:

> Now, to me making this oath fulfilled, and not breaking [it], may it be to share in life and art, being famous according to all men for all time; but [to me] transgressing and forswearing, the opposite of these.

Here, the *Oath* strikes a reader as optimistic, emphasizing the blessings associated with bringing it to completion rather than the (sotto voce) curse attending its violation. Implicitly, the gods invoked at the beginning of the *Oath* serve as the grantors of the fruits of the juror's abiding by the *Oath* while also guaranteeing the opposite. The Greek words here translated "fulfill" literally mean to make something come to its proper goal. By contrast, the verbs opposed to keeping the *Oath* refer to rendering it ineffective, transgressing it, and falsely swearing it. Life, art, and good reputation (among all men and for all time) comprise the (profound) blessings; the opposite, the (grievous) curse. Thus, the *Oath* has a deeply solemn character. The curse for one who violates it proves grave and ominous, validating it as of great import.

Upon this solemn note, the *Oath* concludes. In it we find certain acts singled out as injustices and harms. In sequential order, we have: first, not giving a deadly drug to a patient nor suggesting the same; second (and likewise), not giving a destructive pessary; third, not engaging in sexual acts with anyone upon entering a household; fourth, and finally, not spreading abroad what should not be spoken about, especially that which one learns from the privilege of entering the household, regardless of its connection to therapy. In short, we find the *Oath* singling out killing patients, sexually relating to individuals encountered in one's practice, and violating confidence as acts to be avoided by a physician.

A number of questions concerning these specifically forsworn acts arise. First, are these acts injustices, harms, or corruptions? Second, if so, do they merit the attention they receive? Third, do other signal unmentioned harms deserve notice? We turn to these and allied questions in the next chapter.

Chapter 3
WOUNDING

I n chapter 2 I articulated the *Oath*, which definitively determines the end of medicine as solely therapeutic, excluding wounding. In this chapter, I consider the wounds specifically forsworn in the *Oath*. Because of the (as I shall argue, merited) prominence given to it in the *Oath*, its inherent salience for us mortals, and our corresponding natural interest in medicine's relation to it (e.g., as found in contemporary discussions of physician-assisted suicide—PAS—and euthanasia), in what follows I focus particularly upon the killing of one's patient as the paradigmatic instance of wounding.[1] Needless to say (as the *Oath* itself indicates in its prohibition of sexual relations), a physician can wound by other acts. In keeping with the *Oath*, I also consider wounds other than death among those excluded by Hippocratic medicine. Nonetheless, as dramatically as a corpse differs from a healthy patient, so does killing oppose healing. Accordingly, it archetypically exemplifies wounding. Moreover, as the *Oath* testifies, as history suggests (such as that of the guillotine, examined later), and as contemporary practices indicate (such as PAS, euthanasia, abortion, and attempts to recruit physicians to administer capital punishment), the desire to involve physicians in killing itself has a perennial quality, and therefore it deserves particular attention.

3.1 A DISTINCTION WITHIN THE APOLLONIAN/ASCLEPIAN ACCOUNT

In contrast to the Hippocratic physician, the Apollonian-Asclepian practitioner (first mentioned in 1.3) sees doctoring as entirely consisting of a skill that can be ordered toward the diverse ends of healing or wounding. To this day, this ancient account influences what some understand medicine to be. For, quite simply, it embodies a truth. Namely, that as a skill, technique, or art, medicine can be directed toward opposites—as is the case with arts more generally. (Who is better than the grammarian to write an ungrammatical sentence?) In part because medical know-how makes them good at injuring, physicians themselves occasionally succumb to role-conflation and resort to wounding, even incorporating killing into their overall account of doctoring. Similarly, others who see harming as at times desirable— not limited to, but certainly including patients, their family members, government officials, and those who due to circumstances find injuring useful—attempt to enlist physicians in such acts.

In order to acknowledge noteworthy differences between them, I now propose to distinguish two forms of what I have thus far referred to as the Apollonian/Asclepian account of medicine. I do so in terms of their precise opposition to the Hippocratic account. For while both incorporate killing (and wounding more generally) in their views of medicine, they differ. What I will henceforth call the Apollonian view takes medicine to be a skill oriented toward the health of or injury to the subject. (Shortly, I will contrast wounds compatible with Hippocratic medicine from injuries incompatible with medicine so understood. I realize that I have yet to establish the incompatibility of killing and caring. I will do so in 3.3.1.) While regarding the killing of a patient as an injury to the patient, the Apollonian position does not thereby exclude it from medical practice. By contrast, what I will henceforth call the Asclepian view does exclude outright injury to a patient from medical practice. However, it does not consider the killing of a patient always to be an injury to the patient. Insofar as both include killing within the scope of their practice, they fundamentally oppose the Hippocratic account. To the extent to which they differ in precisely how they incorporate killing, they merit distinction.

While there may not be entirely compelling reasons in the myths concerning Apollo and Asclepius so as to name definitively the accounts as suggested above, it seems fitting to associate with a god that view which appropriates to itself the greatest latitude. For universality seems to be a characteristic of the Apollonian sun (and of divinity more generally). Just as the sun rises on the just and the unjust, without distinction, universally, as it were, so also, the Apollonian physician heals and injures, not observing distinctions between the two.

Moreover (and, perhaps, more to the point for our purposes— for few would regard a physician's injuring without qualification as reasonable), the Apollonian physician will at times injure, even kill a patient (or other individual) insofar as doing so is thought to be less harmful than the available alternatives. Thus, the Apollonian physician will harm outright when doing so putatively reduces overall harm. So, for example, an Apollonian physician may kill his patient when he considers death the least harmful outcome facing the patient. The same, of course, holds for individuals whom we would not call patients (reserving that term for the ill), such as those condemned to death. The Apollonian doctor kills those who would otherwise die more gruesomely. (We will see, e.g., that Dr. Guillotin represents an Apollonian physician in his advocacy of the eponymously named killing machine.) The Apollonian physician's injuring in order to reduce harm assumes a divine character; thus, it is appropriately associated with a god. For it is godlike to make evil produce good, to somehow derive benefit from injury, even if only by injuring to thereby reduce overall harm.

By contrast, the demigod-like Asclepian physician compromises between the divine Apollonian act of outright injury and the mortal Hippocratic exclusion of killing and injury more generally. The Asclepian includes killing (and thus acts somewhat divinely) while proposing that it is not injurious, but, rather, beneficial (and thus acts as a mortal who does not attempt to bring good from evil). Thus, the Asclepian doctor, like Asclepius himself, has a half-god-like character. By the above, I hope to indicate that decent grounds exist for so naming these accounts. Having named the diverse accounts, I will now argue that one can distinguish wounds compatible with medicine as exclusively therapeutic from those, Apollonian or Asclepian, not compatible—particularly the killing of one's patient.

3.2 COMING TO TERMS: DISTINGUISHING WOUNDS FROM INJURIES

As noted in discussion of wounds of incision (in 1.2), healing itself does not entirely exclude wounding. It does not necessarily prohibit even gross wounds; indeed, it may require such wounds. At one extreme, consider amputation of a gangrenous limb (an ancient practice described in the Hippocratic text *On Joints*)—certainly, a profound wound. More prosaically, a therapeutic interaction with a physician eventually and characteristically involves a warning that "this will hurt." One surmises that physicians have been saying that since the dawn of medicine and shall do so for as long as the sick seek care. Routine medical practices—sticking with needles, drawing blood, cutting into, even the pain associated with anesthetizing prior to such cutting—suggest the difficulty of distinguishing healing from wounding. Excellent healing at times requires cutting, burning, and even amputating.

In order to support the claim that physicians ought to avoid conflating the role of healer with that of wounder, one must adequately distinguish healing from wounding. Clearly, given the necessity of cutting, burning, etc., wounding in itself does not make one a wounder in contrast to a healer. Can one distinguish the wounding that partially constitutes healing from that the performance of which would render one a wounder *sans phrase* so as to contrast exclusively caregiving (Hippocratic) medicine from the duo of Apollonian or Asclepian medical technique? To this task I now turn with the goal of arguing to kill one's patient, even at that patient's request, is to injure one's patient and, thereby, to conflate the opposed roles of healer and wounder.

A preliminary difficulty concerns terms. How ought we speak of these two distinct, yet easily confused phenomena? That is, wounding that comports with medical acts ordered toward health and wounding that does not. Thus far I have contrasted the healer from the wounder, suggesting that we might contrast healing from wounding. This, however, does not serve. For, as noted, excellent care at times requires wounding. Indeed, part of doctoring involves wound care, which includes the care of wounds that physicians needfully inflict on their patients in treating them.

Because medicine itself speaks of wounds as part and parcel of essential medical care, I will contrast what I have thus far referred to generically as wounding from the more specific form of wounding that purposefully injures (in which the wounder deals). I do so with a view to claiming that Hippocratic (or exclusively therapeutic) medicine does not necessarily exclude wounding and wounds, while it does necessarily exclude injuring-wounds and injuries. (Henceforth, I will use "injury" to refer to injuring-wounds.) Indeed, in the *Oath* the juror swears to keep the sick free from all injury (literally, the deleterious). While somewhat stipulative, in addition to comporting with the *Oath*, this usage agrees with the way contemporary physicians actually speak. That is, a doctor characteristically tells a patient how to care for wounds the physician inflicted (e.g., incisions, stitches, and cauterizations) while not speaking of how to care for injuries (what

I here specify as wounding-injuries) the physician visited upon the patient. This, of course, does not mean that physicians do not injure their patients. Indeed, errors amount to inadvertent injuries. It does mean, however, that in the practice of Hippocratic or solely caregiving medicine, injuring a patient amounts to, at best, an error and, at worst, the abandonment of medicine entailed by the adoption of the role of deliberate wounder. (The wounder wounds on purpose, delivering injuring-wounds. The healer heals on purpose. Of course, we name both by what they do deliberately.) With these terms in place, I now turn to the work of showing how the realities they name actually differ such that excellent solely caregiving (Hippocratic) medicine includes wounds of therapy while excluding the specific injury of killing found in both Apollonian and Asclepian technique. At the end of this chapter I will consider the other injuries of sexual exploitation and gossip which the *Oath* specifically excludes.

3.3 HIPPOCRATIC MEDICINE DISTINGUISHED FROM APOLLONIAN AND ASCLEPIAN SKILL

In distinguishing Hippocratic medicine from the various techniques that admit of killing, there are three difficulties. First, and most generally, how does one practically—and not simply terminologically, as I have thus far done—distinguish wounds from injuries? Second, and more specifically, does the killing of one's patient always count as an injury? Obviously in the *Oath*, the patient asking the physician for a deadly drug appears, along Asclepian lines, not to regard this as an injury—or, taking an Apollonian approach, acknowledges it to be harmful, but the least harmful of a number of other unpalatable options. Similarly, contemporary advocates of PAS and euthanasia (and practitioners who assist patient-suicides or euthanize) regard such practices either as positively beneficial (Asclepian) or as the least injurious alternative confronting the patient (Apollonian).

This brings us to our third difficulty, perhaps the greatest. Namely, does doctoring necessarily exclude injuring? Consider. An Apollonian advocate of euthanasia or PAS might agree that the patient's death injures the patient while also maintaining that a physician should so injure the patient because it is the least injurious harm that the patient will suffer. Thus, as an instance of reducing the harm one's patient will suffer, perhaps it comports with medicine's orientation toward healing? Further afield, yet still along Apollonian lines, some maintain that physicians should participate in capital punishment insofar as, by killing well, they reduce the condemned person's distress. To consider an even more extreme case, while acknowledging that torturing an individual injures the individual, one might think that physicians should do this because they could do it with the least injury to the victim. While a jarring proposal, one finds physician participation in torture seriously proposed—indeed practiced, with due infamy, as Miles 2006 and Lauritzen 2013 attest.

In response to the above-noted three issues, I argue three points. First, that one can in practice distinguish wounds from injuries. Second, that killing necessarily injures. Third, that once one identifies acts that necessarily injure, one can argue that such acts are, thereby, incompatible with the role of caregiver, even when undertaken along Apollonian lines to reduce overall harm. Simply put, caring, while it need not exclude wounding, necessarily excludes injuring.[2] In other words, therapeutically "first, do no harm" holds. One who injures— even thereby to reduce injury—can no longer purport to be a mender, healer, caregiver, physician, doctor, or therapeutic professional. Let us now turn to the first task of practically and not just terminologically distinguishing wounds from injuries.

Amputation instances a profound, gross, extreme wound. For by it, in addition to cutting and burning, an organ is forever removed from the organism. I here use "organ" (from Greek *organon*, meaning "tool") somewhat liberally (yet consonant with our more restrictive use of it) to refer to a distinct part of the organism which fulfills a task or function, as does a tool. Amputation removes a tool from the organism (a system of tools ordered toward an overarching goal, the flourishing—literally, the flowering or bearing of fruit—of the being to which they belong). To amputate is to maim, mutilate, partially to destroy the organism as such. That is, to remove an organ (a tool whose unique function contributes to the overall well-being of the entity) deeply assaults the organism in its organic character and not simply as superficially vulnerable (in the literal sense of being woundable, from the Latin *vulnus*, meaning "wound").

As the removal of an organ, amputation illustrates a permanent diminishment of the whole. By contrast, when a dermatologist removes cancerous skin cells, although she cuts and cauterizes, she need not permanently alter the organism in its integrity of organs. Certainly, cutting and burning, she leaves a scar and, thereby, forever mars the skin of the patient, perhaps for all to see. Nevertheless, the organic whole remains. The amputee, however, loses an integral part of the integrated whole. The removal of a toe, a leg, a finger, an arm, a breast, a spleen, or an appendix vitiates the entity's integrity. It is no longer intact, no longer whole, no longer complete.

Accordingly, if one can differentiate amputation from injuring, one will have advanced well along the path in contrasting wounds (compatible with healing) from injuries (incompatible with healing). For, given the thorough character of wounding that amputation instances, the criteria by which amputation counts as healing will capture less profound instances of wounding exemplified by the incision and burning found in amputation. In short, if we can make the case for categorizing the maiming and mutilating found in amputation as healing, we will have discerned how wounding differs from injuring.

So, what of amputating? A reader understandably may find the following answer anticlimactic, because (I suggest) it is intuitively correct. Although a profound wound, amputation falls within the boundaries of excellent, caregiving, entirely therapeutic, Hippocratic medicine (and, needless to say, of current sound medical practice). When the part jeopardizes the whole, the part ought to be severed from the whole. We amputate the part for the sake of the remaining whole, whose welfare constitutes the part's point and purpose. As is the case with any organ, one finds the good of the leg in the good of the organism to which it belongs. Threatening that good with a deadly infection, the part must be sacrificed for the remaining whole on behalf of which it exists in the first place. Thus, amputation, although permanently marring, wounding, and maiming does not ultimately make the organism worse off than it would otherwise be—namely, dead. More generally, while a wound mars, blemishes, diminishes the good of the whole, it fundamentally serves the whole's good, in this case, the health of the organism. By contrast, an injury leaves the organism worse off, impairs, and proves deleterious to the organism. Thus, a medical wound serves the whole's good, while an injury does not. Needless to say, the patient benefited by medical wounds and harmed by injuries instances the relevant organic whole.

With the distinction between wounds and injuries in place, let us turn to our second question. Namely, is, as the *Oath* proposes, the killing of one's patient at the request of the patient always an injury to the patient? On the face of things, killing is bad, to be avoided, injurious. Of course, so also are acts such as cutting, burning, and amputating. In accord with the Asclepian viewpoint, can death at times be a wound inflicted for the good of the whole and not an injury (as is the case with a therapeutic amputation)? Alternatively (and this instances our third previously noted question), if death constitutes an injury, can one along Apollonian lines inflict it as least injurious and, therefore, done with a view to the overall welfare of the patient killed?

3.3.1 The Asclepian Account Disputed

First, consider the Asclepian account that death at times benefits the patient. Obviously, the *Oath* rejects such a killing. Yet, if the subject to be killed desires death, what reasons can the physician offer for not killing? Clearly, the injury is not to be found in the frustration of the patient's desire for continued life when it is the patient who requests to be killed. How, precisely, is it an injury?

While presumably not always an injustice (e.g., legitimate killing in defense of self or others), death always injures the one who dies. Indeed, it constitutes the terminus of all diseases and what all injuries intimate, the final, last assault one can suffer. As the Greek word for the ill (*kamnontes*) itself suggests in its dual reference to the sick (those who are laboring) and to the dead (those who have labored), sickness ends in death. In dying, the sick one falls for the last time. By death the ill one becomes, literally, a cadaver, "one fallen," a corpse, defunct, deceased, dead.

Indeed, "injury" does not adequately capture the harm that death instances. One suffers an injury; characteristically, one undergoes, endures, and survives injury. Indeed, for these and allied reasons, we do not speak of death as merely an injury. Death undoes, dissolves, annihilates the subject. Death ends even the possibility of undergoing injury. The sick labor under a burden; medicine attempts to alleviate that burden. To undo the subject by killing him does not lift the burden. Rather, to do so is to take the side of illness against the patient by unwinding him. The death-dealer does disease's last work.

Of course (as the above-noted Greek word for the ill itself suggests), death does end the labor of the sick. For this reason, some understandably (albeit mistakenly) suggest that killing comports with medical practice. For medicine attempts to lessen dis-ease. Death goes one better than medicine by permanently ending one's susceptibility to illness. Medicine's essential activity, however, does not concern ending sickness, but, rather, caring for patients who labor under disease. Simply put, one cannot care for another by destroying that other, even at his request. Therapy, caring for a subject, requires the subject to exist so that he may receive one's care.

Of woe, destruction, ruin, and decay, the worst is death: woe-full, all-destroying, utterly ruinous, and, ultimately, our rotting. Because killing completely ruins the one killed, medicine cannot admit killing and remain therapeutic. Caregiving and killing mutually exclude one another. Therefore, a physician cannot give care by killing. The killing healer abandons medicine. In killing he cannot claim to offer therapy. Because caregiving defines doctoring, he no longer practices medicine.

Killing performed by a doctor is oxymoronic, a practical contradiction. To boil a lamb in its mother's milk is perverse, a twisting of the way things ought to be. For the ewe has milk to sustain the lambkin. So also, a mender's killing a patient goes against the physician's raison d'être. Namely, to help the sick fare as well as they can. Killing by caregivers always incorporates dis-order, wrongness, what is not due, or injustice, even when practiced on those who, otherwise, ought to be killed (e.g., if one accepts capital punishment as, in principle, justifiable).

Allow that the above serves as a reasonable response to the Asclepian claim that death does not always injure a patient. What of the Apollonian position that acknowledges that death injures, but that sometimes it amounts to a less injurious harm than that confronting the patient and, therefore, comports with caregiving as a reduction of harm? The Apollonian account suffers from the defect afflicting the Asclepian while in one respect being more attractive. While it shares the fatal Asclepian flaw of attempting to incorporate killing into caring, it does not do so by denying the primal truth that death injures the one killed. Rather, the Apollonian physician acknowledges that to kill is to injure while proposing that since greater injuries than death at the hands of a skilled physician confront some individuals—for example, a more grisly death—in order to lessen the injury, a doctor would do well to deal death.

However, and here I repeat myself, just as a fireman does not preserve a house by burning it down to the ground, so also a physician does not care for a patient (or anyone else, for that matter) by killing him, even if by doing so the patient (or subject) dies less grimly. Killing practically contradicts therapy. Putatively, such killing has aspects of compassion, sympathy, tender-heartedness, and mercy (in the way in which the executioner's final blow may be accurately spoken of as a coup de grace—literally, a grace-stroke, a blow of mercy). Regardless, it cannot be therapy. For it destroys the sick. Among apparently compassionate, sympathetic, tender-hearted, and merciful acts, physicians, as physicians, must limit themselves to those acts that have the sine qua non feature of not rendering caring impossible.

Some might think it entirely theoretical to entertain the Apollonian account. For once one broadly argues, as I have, against the compatibility of killing and caring, need one consider the specific case of killing less injuriously? Does it not fall under the more general prohibition? Indeed, it does. However, because some appear to find the Apollonian position more compelling than the Asclepian, I treat of it separately. Thinkers do so in part because in some respect it makes more sense of medicine conceived of as a mere technique than does the Asclepian view. For, as previously noted, practitioners of the medical technique can kill well. If the thing to be done well is in itself not objectionable, is it not better that it be done well than done poorly? This apparently reasonable attitude underlies notable instances of the desire to have physicians kill, along Apollonian lines. When some doctors see others killing (presumably) justly but badly—i.e., with avoidable distress and suffering—they understandably may (albeit somewhat officiously) take it upon themselves to do a better job, as it were. Alternatively, others (e.g., legislators—in 3.3.3 we will consider contemporary attempts to involve physicians in capital punishment) might propose that physicians kill. For they will no doubt kill both well (technically) and more successfully than others lacking a medical education.

3.3.2 Apollonian Killing Considered: Dr. Guillotin and his "Simple Mechanism"

To see how physicians might involve themselves in the Apollonian project of harm-reductive killing, consider the origin of the guillotine, one of history's most infamous means of killing. The legacy of a number of physicians (Dr. Guillotin and his contemporary the surgeon Antoine Louis), it exemplifies how doctors can become preoccupied with killing well, contradicting their vocation exclusively to care. I offer it as a cautionary tale lest a reader take the Apollonian account to be largely fanciful.

Prerevolutionary France reserved decapitation by sword-stroke at the hands of an executioner to the nobility and those of high social status, the presumption in part being that a person of good birth would have the "firmness to stand the trial"—in the words of Charles Henry Sanson, Paris' executioner at Guillotin's time (Ainsworth 1863, 273)—while one of base birth would not.[3] Certainly, the soon-to-be-decapitated victim needed fortitude to remain still while kneeling lest the sword blade glance off his or her neck. By contrast, commoners were typically hanged.[4] In this context, Dr. Guillotin comes upon the scene.

Legend has it that the pregnant *Mme*. Guillotin took to her bed of labor after a walk during which she chanced to see a condemned criminal undergo the ordeal of the wheel. The wheel—also called the Catherine wheel after Saint Catherine who was reputedly martyred on such a device in fourth-century Alexandria—was Procrustean in the worst way. The victim was laid upon and affixed to the cartwheel with wedges and ropes. The executioner then broke the bones of her arms and legs with an iron bar. Sometimes the bones were broken with a view to threading the soon-to-be corpse within the wheel's spokes for subsequent displaying. The executioner's coup de grâce put the victim out of her misery.

Regardless of the veracity of the legend, Joseph-Ignace Guillotin was born on May 28, 1738. He went on to become the physician whose name to this day calls to mind mechanized capital punishment. As Victor Hugo notes:

> There are unlucky men; Christopher Columbus is not able to
> attach his name to his discovery; Guillotin is not able to detach
> his from his invention. (author's translation, Hugo 1976, 299)[5]

While Guillotin left no (other) progeny, legend also has it that the family—failing in their request that the infamous machine no longer be called *la guillotine*—went on to change their own name, to what we are not told (Kershaw 1993, 10).

On the oft-noted issue of Guillotine's name being assimilated to that of the machine, one notes that Roederer, the *procureur général syndic* (comparable to a US district attorney) who solicited proposals from craftsmen for such items considered the bid submitted by the customarily used contractor Guidon too high. When queried, Guidon responded that his workmen demanded enormous wages "from a prejudice against the object in view." Roederer responded:

> the prejudice, indeed, exists; but I have offers from other per-
> sons to undertake the work, provided they should not be asked
> to sign contracts, or in any other way to have their names
> exposed as connected with the object. (Guillotin 1844, 220)

Clearly, in the spring of 1792, Parisian carpenters were willing to build a decapitating machine, but wanted no nominal part in the project.

While Guillotin initially proposed "my machine" ("*ma machine*"), the surgeon Antoine Louis played a much larger role in designing the actual mechanism. Experimenting on human cadavers, Dr. Louis found that the diagonal blade better severed tissue (Weiner 1972, 85). In recognition of his role in designing the French version (for there had been numerous others contemporaneously and in previous centuries), for a short period of time the device received the names *La Louisette* and *La Louison*.

Events, however, forever link the *simple mécanisme* to Guillotin, whose name, ironically, numbers him among the most famous physicians in history—although not for a properly medical advance. Perhaps looming largest among the fate-filled contingencies by which the mechanism was named is the fact that, in French, *machine* rhymes with *guillotine* (the feminine form of *Guillotin*). Indeed, the Chevalier de Champcenetz, who on July 23, 1794, would die under a guillotine, so baptized the device in a topical song *(couplets de circonstance)* set to the popular minuet by the composer André-Joseph Exaudet *(du menuet d'Exaudet)*:

> *La machine/Qui 'simplement' nous tuera/Et que l'on nommera/Guillotine!* [The Machine / which 'simply' will kill us / And to which we will give the name / Guillotine!] (Pellet 1873, 163)[6]

"*Simplement*" here refers to Dr. Guillotin's too irresistible "*simple mécanisme*," a phrase found in his initial proposal, which we now consider.

Egalitarianism coupled with a humanitarian Enlightenment-based faith in mechanization in contrast to the presumably too-often-proved messiness of manual killing (including sword-stroke beheadings) apparently moved Guillotin to propose mechanical decapitation as the sole means of imposing the death penalty. On October 10, 1789, as a delegate to the French National Assembly, Dr. Guillotin proposed a bill of six articles reforming the penal system of *l'ancien regime*. The relevant article read:

> The method of punishment shall be the same for all persons on whom the law shall pronounce a sentence of death, whatever the crime of which they are guilty. The criminal shall be decapitated. Decapitation is to be effected by a simple mechanism. (Arasse 1989, 11)

The record indicates that the revolutionary penal reform did not receive discussion on that day. Rather, on December 1, 1789, it was reconsidered. Dr. Guillotin spoke on its behalf. At one point in the discussion, Guillotin enthusiastically said something along the lines of "with my machine I strike off your head in the blinking of an eye and without your feeling the least pain."[7]

These words were met with an immense outburst of laughter. Of course, as numerous historians note, while such machines already existed—indeed, predated Dr. Guillotin's much-noted proposal by centuries—he himself did not have such a mechanism. The eponymous version would not exist until three years had passed since the fateful proposal of October 1789.

Guillotin's infamous declaration came in response to a concern articulated by Jean-Sifrein Maury (admitted to the French Academy in 1785):

> the Abbé Maury, with prophetic sagacity, objected to the adoption of decapitation as a general punishment, "because it

might tend to deprave the people by *familiarizing them with the sight of blood"* [*"la décapitation n'aurait-elle point pour effet de dépraver le peuple, en la familiarisant avec la vue du sang?"*]; but Maury's objection seems to have made no great impression at a time when no one—not even the sagacious and eloquent Abbé himself—could have foreseen such a prodigality of legal murders—such a deluge of blood as afterwards afforded so practical and so frightful a corroboration of his theoretical suggestion. (Croker 1853, 11, original emphasis)

The exchange must have been funny to witness: on the one side the fusty Abbé; on the other, the progressive Enlightenment physician. As noted, the scenario ends with "a great outburst of laughter" (*"un immense éclat de rire"*) when *le médecin* takes the Apollonian approach. Dr. Guillotin aspired, along harm-minimizing lines and in keeping with egalitarian values, to reduce executions to a coup de grâce delivered by his *"simple mécanisme."*

Did Guillotin and Louis err as physicians by becoming so involved in, respectively, proposing and developing a means of capital punishment? Certainly. Indeed, spontaneous laughter, ridicule, and the humorous ditties directed at Guillotin rely, quite simply as humor does, upon the laughable, ludicrous, ridiculous conjunction of a doctor killing, apparently enthusiastically. Doctors care; killing destroys. Laughter arises reasonably from one thinking about the incongruity of a physician eagerly killing.

In advancing this judgment, I concede that the guillotine (presumably) reduces the distress of the condemned. Needless to say, this is good. Further, and for the sake of considering a physician's involvement in capital punishment, let us stipulate that the death penalty can be administered justly. That is, that such a punishment is not inherently wrong. Well then, what of it? Why should Drs. Guillotin and Louis not, respectively, propose and develop this more humane means of killing those condemned to death?

I will argue shortly that there are numerous further reasons in virtue of which physicians ought not to kill or assist in the killing of their patients, some of which also bear on this more specific question of capital punishment. Here, however, I want briefly to note a reason more relevant to this specific issue. Namely, that those condemned to death do not suffer from an illness. In other words, to render capital punishment more humane is not to treat a patient. The patient serves as the ineliminable, necessary, sine qua non subject of a physician's ministrations. Absent a patient, the healer lacks the one for whom doctoring cares. A patient, as previously noted, labors under an illness. By contrast, one condemned to death does not. Admirable as it may be to reduce the distress of one so condemned, for a physician to do so by becoming intimately involved in killing doubly disorients medicine from its focus upon both exclusively caring and doing so for those laboring under a disease.

While it might strike a reader as a somewhat quaint description, Drs. Guillotin and Louis act officiously in devoting their energies to perfecting the administration of the death penalty. That is, they amount to well-intentioned meddlers. The earnest Guillotin and Louis over-eagerly offer their uncalled-for services and take upon themselves, as if it were a duty, the improvement of killing. Ironically, they do so with respect to the very opposite of their actual medical office to care for a patient's health. Not only did they fail to mind their own (noble) calling to heal the sick, perhaps a venial fault, but they also acted perversely with respect to it, presumably a graver failing.

Dr. Bourru eulogized Guillotin, his friend and fellow physician. The surname "Bourru" means "rough" in French. Moreover, in the context of the guillotine the name suggests *le bourreau*, the public executioner—from the French verb *bourrer*, meaning "to strike." This confirms Hugo's apt observation previously noted; Guillotin remains unlucky. (Or, perhaps, he receives his historic due?) For even in his eulogy the very name of the man who offers it cannot but remind us of the infamous machine. Apparently obtuse to certain details concerning his subject's history, Dr. Bourru speaks as follows:

> Unfortunately for our colleague his philanthropic gesture [*motion*, can one help but think of the blade repeatedly falling?], which was approved and bore fruit [*donné*] in an instrument to which the populace [*le vulgaire*] has appended his name, made him many enemies. How true it is that it is difficult to benefit mankind [*de faire du bien aux hommes*] without some unpleasantness resulting for oneself. (Arasse 1989, English translation, 9; Arasse 1987, French original, 18)

Here, the well-named Dr. Bourru roughly observes the Latin advice respecting the dead—*non nisi bonum*: speak nothing but good. One wonders, however, if the truth does not suffer. Certainly, euphemism triumphs. Improved killing is a philanthropic gesture. The vulgar are charged with appending his name to what Guillotin himself first declared as "*ma machine*." Yet, conversely, we are told that the unjustly named machine is a gift, the fruit (*donné*) of the gesture. To compound matters, he ends with the sanctimonious observation that it is difficult to do good to men without some unpleasantness to oneself. One asks: just how hard is it for a competent physician of middling character to do good to his fellow human beings by minding his own business, namely, by caring for their health? Moreover, does a philanthropist make many enemies in virtue of his actual philanthropy? Enough. Guillotin was a misguided busybody who became involved in precisely the business that he as a physician should have last been involved in: the perfection of killing. Presumably, his name shall (duly) remain infamous. For our purposes, he illustrates the error of the Apollonian physician.

3.3.3 Attempts to Make Physicians Apollonian

Guillotin exemplifies the Apollonian physician who proposes to kill less harmfully. Corresponding to the Apollonian physician, one finds a public requesting that doctors kill. Recall the words of the anthropologist Margaret Mead (noted previously in 1.3). She writes:

> society is always attempting to make the physician into a
> killer—to kill the defective child at birth, to leave the sleeping

pills beside the bed of the cancer patient, ... it is the duty of society to protect the physician from such requests. (Levine 1972, 324-5)

Mead observes that we repeatedly ask physicians to kill. I wish, briefly, to note that our attempts do not seem to have flagged.

One finds contemporary governments asking physicians (and allied caregivers such as nurses and pharmacists) to be significantly involved in capital punishment. Indeed, some governments even require that the death penalty include a physician's extensive participation. In the United States, the state of North Carolina mandates that physicians and nurses (and, by implication, pharmacists) participate closely in carrying out the death penalty (in contrast to cooperating in an incidental fashion by, e.g., a doctor certifying death). The Supreme Court of North Carolina ruled that the North Carolina Medical Board (which licenses physicians) cannot restrict physician participation in capital punishment to the physician being physically present at an execution. Rather, in opposition to the Medical Board's (on the face of things, principled and balanced) stance, the legislature can, as it did in North Carolina General Statute 15-190, require that a physician "monitor the essential body functions of the condemned inmate and notify the Warden immediately upon his or her determination that the inmate shows signs of undue pain or suffering."

Notably, the legislature decrees that the physician be employed lest undue pain and suffering in the administration of the death penalty render the same a violation of the US Constitution's eighth amendment, prohibiting "cruel and unusual punishment." This instances an Apollonian view of the physician as a harm-reducer. So conceived, one would naturally enlist a physician so as to punish least harmfully. Of course, this account of medicine errs. For it proposes that punishing (which necessarily involves the imposition of a harm) comports with medicine. Yet, medicine exclusively cares for a subject. Moreover, it avoids harming, especially deliberate harming—even in order to reduce overall harm. Additionally, as noted, one mistakenly thinks of the condemned as a proper subject of the physician's therapy (or the subject of medical caregivers more generally—nurses and pharmacists). Caregivers administer to patients, those laboring under illness. While dire, being condemned to death does not make one a patient. Thus, those who would have caregivers punish stray widely.

Referring to the incompatibility of punishing and medicine, the North Carolina Medical Board (in its prohibition of a physician's so monitoring the condemned) noted that "physician participation in capital punishment is a departure from the ethics of the medical profession" (N. C. 2009, 645). Additionally, the Medical Board cited the American Medical Association's Code of Medical Ethics section 2.06, which distinguishes the personal opinion of the medical practitioner concerning the morality of the death penalty from the ethic of a member of a profession "dedicated to preserving life when there is hope of doing so" (N. C. 2009, 645). The American Medical Association acknowledges that the profession has a therapeutic ethic that prohibits a physician from cooperating in imposing the death penalty, regardless of the justice (or lack thereof) of capital punishment.

Tortuously, the court opined that since capital punishment was not a medical procedure, the Medical Board lacked jurisdiction to prevent physicians from participating in it. By this convoluted logic, the Medical Board's authority would extend no further than regulating actual medical procedures, having no ability to forbid physicians from doing acts deemed not to be appropriately medical. It would be as ludicrous to tell the court that it must limit itself to regulating constitutional acts, since unconstitutional acts are, well, frankly, not constitutional and, thereby, not subject to a court that attends to what is constitutional. Of course, just as regulating what is legal involves one in regulating the illegal (by, e.g., forbidding and punishing it), so too regulating what is medical involves one in regulating what is not medical. Certainly, the category not medical is too broad, including as it does everything that is not medical, such as an interest in abstract art. The relevant set of acts that the court as a court or the medical board as a medical board appropriately oversees concerns those that are specifically opposed to law or medicine, namely, the illegal or (for want of a better word) the immedical in the sense of contrary to medicine. When the medical board forbids physicians from using their regulated medical skill to kill those to be capitally punished, it makes a judgment concerning what violates the regulated use of the skill. Were it, for example, to forbid physicians from advocating for (or against) capital punishment, it would overstep its proper bounds. Such advocacy is not itself an exercise of the medical skill; thus, it falls outside the purview of the board.

Given our apparent propensity to suborn physicians in killing, Hippocrates does well to forswear killing. Previously, I noted that one finds many reasons for doctors to avoid killing. Allow me now to turn to such considerations.

3.4 FURTHER REASONS WHY PHYSICIANS OUGHT NOT KILL

Say the above is the case, what further reasons besides the profound injury it instances can one offer for a physician's refraining from killing a patient? A physician's killing of a patient, as is the case with other egregious acts, produces overdetermined wrongness.[8] It instances myriad bad characteristics. Consider a few of the more obvious.

First, by killing the sick, the physician dramatically undermines the trust patients needfully place in their physicians. Moreover, physicians thereby render ambiguous the deaths of patients that do at times occur in the normal practice of medicine. Consider the following famous story found in Plutarch's life of Alexander the Great. Plutarch recounts Alexander's profound trust in his physician who, as the story indicates, personally ran great risks in treating Alexander:

> it was sickness that detained him [Alexander the Great] there, which some say he contracted from his fatigues, others from bathing in the river Cydnus, whose waters were exceedingly cold. However it happened, none of his physicians would venture to give him any remedies, they thought his case so desperate, and were so afraid of the suspicions and ill-will of the Macedonians if they should fail in the cure; till Philip, the Acarnanian, seeing how critical his case was, but relying

on his own well-known friendship for him, resolved to try the last efforts of his art, and rather hazard his own credit and life than suffer him to perish for want of physic, which he confidently administered to him, encouraging him to take it boldly, if he desired a speedy recovery, in order to prosecute the war. At this very time, Parmenio wrote to Alexander from the camp, bidding him have a care of Philip, as one who was bribed by Darius to kill him, with great sums of money, and a promise of his daughter in marriage. When he had perused the letter, he put it under his pillow, without showing it so much as to any of his most intimate friends, and when Philip came in with the potion, he took it with great cheerfulness and assurance, giving him meantime the letter to read. This was a spectacle well worth being present at, to see Alexander take the draught and Philip read the letter at the same time, and then turn and look upon one another, but with different sentiments; for Alexander's looks were cheerful and open, to show his kindness to and confidence in his physician, while the other was full of surprise and alarm at the accusation, appealing to the gods to witness his innocence, sometimes lifting up his hands to heaven, and then throwing himself down by the bedside, and beseeching Alexander to lay aside all fear, and follow his directions without apprehension. For the medicine at first worked so strongly as to drive, so to say, the vital forces into the interior; he lost his speech, and falling into a swoon, had scarce any sense or pulse left. However, in no long time, by Philip's means, his health and strength returned, and he showed himself in public to the Macedonians, who were in continual fear and dejection until they saw him abroad again. (Plutarch 1992, 153–4)[9]

Regardless of one's worldly stature, as a vulnerable patient one must trust one's physician—even Alexander the Great must do so. Indeed, Alexander seems well aware of this necessity. Yet, were medical practitioners on record as open to killing, upon what grounds could one base such confidence in one's doctor not to kill? Moreover, as suggested by the hesitancy of the other physicians to treat Alexander lest they be held responsible for an untoward outcome, physicians themselves benefit when others know that they forswear killing a patient. Additionally, note how in this vignette, therapeutic treatment can at times appear to be lethal. Confidence that a physician will not kill aids one to undergo such care. A patient sure of his physician's professional commitment not to kill can put to the side the added anxiety that accompanies wondering whether one's caregiver might take one's life. Simply put, were doctors not to forswear killing, patients' trust in physicians would be less both forthcoming and merited.

Second, by assisting in the suicide of or killing a terminally ill sick person who wants death due to loss of autonomy (the most common contemporary justification for physician-assisted suicide and euthanasia), the physician medicalizes existential, not psychosomatic distress (the proper object of therapy). Indeed, the physician would thereby emphatically answer Hamlet's question by asserting "'tis nobler to end the sea of troubles" called life. This is hardly a medically indicated response; indeed, "to be or not to be?" is not a medical question, but rather one that arises in the tumultuous waters in which we humans find ourselves. Doctors appropriately treat patients suffering from diseases and allied symptoms: cancer, diabetes, arthritis, pain, dementia, dyspnea, nausea, vomiting, incontinence, and failure of heart, kidney, liver, lungs, and so on, and on, and on. For these instance disease and the distress attendant upon disease. To lack control over one's bladder is to suffer from a disorder aptly addressed by a physician. To lack control over the time and manner of one's death partially defines the human condition. To regard this lack as a disease in need of a healer's treatment errs fundamentally. For one thereby treats mortality—the "blight man was born for" —as if it were a medical problem soluble by sterile technique instead of that at which the mind appropriately boggles.

Third, by so responding to a patient's request to be killed (or assisted in self-killing), the physician jeopardizes the welfare of vulnerable others, rendering them, too, susceptible to this injury. Consider two such representative individuals: first, a patient similar to the one assisted or killed by the physician; second, a suicidal person.

A patient similarly situated to the one whom the physician aided in self-killing (or killed in euthanasia) numbers among the vulnerable. How will the individual laboring under the same disease come to regard the continuance of his own therapy upon learning that his ill peer requested death and his physician assisted in its deliverance or delivered it? Given the momentousness of either assisting in killing or killing, the physician cannot assert that he did so simply because that is what the patient wanted. No. The physician must consider the assisting or the killing as justified by the relevant disease. Moreover, the physician must be thought by reasonable others so to regard the killing. That is, the patient in those circumstances who wanted to be killed by self or others had good reason in the physician's considered judgment. By killing or assisting in the killing of a patient, a physician indicates to reasonable others that having that disorder is a good reason to be killed by one's self or others. Thus, from the participating physician's perspective, a comparable patient has good reason to kill himself (or be killed). This judgment inferred from the physician's act of killing (or assisting in killing) amounts to a further burden the ill must carry. Slightly further afield, consider a suicidal individual.

By assisting a patient's suicide or by euthanizing a patient, a doctor suggests that killing solves human trials and tribulations. Desperate people such as the suicidal—to take but one cohort of those who labor under a burden—seek such clear-cut answers to seemingly insurmountable problems. If endorsed by physicians, killing—usually recognized as a pessimistic, unimaginative, and simplistic answer to a conundrum—will seem to many unstably perched on ledges to be an insightful response. We the many—fortunately not being suicidal—chronically fail to realize how ambivalent toward death one is who is suicidal. We tend to think one who recurs to suicide must be bent on the same. For, we ask incredulously: "who would kill herself were she not committed to her own demise?" Yet, as too many realize only after another's suicide, even the most offhand request not to kill one's self can serve as an adequate reason not do so for one who otherwise would. How will a suicidal person fare if, of all professionals, a physician recommends as therapeutic, prescribes, and participates in the killing of a patient?[10] Concern for the vulnerable argues against physician involvement in patient-killing.

Fourth, and allied to the above point regarding similarly situated patients, recourse to killing will retard the development of medicine as an art. Removing one of the boundaries within which the physician labors will not lead to new ways of healing the sick. Rather, it will impede the advancement of medicine as therapeutic. For, if one adequate response to a specific disease is to kill the patient who bears the disorder, why try to develop therapies for that illness? One has a putatively effective therapy: patient-killing.[11] Restraint from killing patients will tend to advance the development of therapies to treat the very diseases on account of which one would otherwise kill them.[12] Medicine advances within limits—as is the case with practices more generally.

Fifth and finally, by killing even in a putatively therapeutic manner, the physician undermines medicine's ability not to be suborned into killing more generally and for diverse purposes. By orienting the skill toward acts profoundly deleterious to those subject to them, the physician invites requests for other harmful uses of the skill, such as administering capital punishment, torture, and waging war. Once physicians themselves disorient their own art from exclusively caring, they subject themselves as artists to further disorientation by others. Presumably, those others will show less sensitivity to concerns native to physicians, such as the welfare of the subject upon whom one practices. But, then again, those others may find the (Asclepian or Apollonian) physician's own account of how killing comports with caring of questionable subtlety.

At this point in the discussion, some will wonder if a physician must not kill, does this entail that a doctor must do everything to keep a patient alive? If a physician abides by the Hippocratic prohibition against euthanasia and physician-assisted suicide, does he thereby commit himself to not allowing a patient to die if he can prevent her death? For example, in a modern medical context, may a Hippocratic physician forgo the use of or remove a currently employed medical intervention when so doing results in the patient's death? To take but one such intervention, would a physician violate the Hippocratic prohibition either by not employing a ventilator or by removing a patient from a ventilator when by so doing the patient will expire? Moreover, what of the apparently more difficult case (as a causing of death and not an allowing to die) often referred to as terminal sedation? In such a case (rare but not unheard-of at the end of life), the patient's agitation by pain cannot be treated short of sedating the patient to such an extent that he stops breathing or breathes inadequately to sustain life. How could this not amount to a violation of the Hippocratic prohibition? Yet, if it does, then the Hippocratic physician would appear to be handicapped as a caregiver. For his acceptance of the prohibition against killing his patient will prevent him from treating his patient's distress at otherwise intractable pain at the end of life. Let us address these challenges to the Hippocratic prohibition against killing one's patient.

3.5 IF THOU SHALT NOT KILL MUST ONE STRIVE OFFICIOUSLY TO KEEP ALIVE?

As noted, two distinct yet allied scenarios confront the physician who acknowledges the import of the Hippocratic prohibition against giving a deadly drug to a patient or suggesting the same. First, we have the issue of allowing a patient to die. Second, we have presumably the more problematic case of actually causing the patient's death as a concomitant of relieving her agitation in the face of intractable pain. Consider allowing first.

In the humorous poem *The Latest Decalogue*, the Victorian poet A. H. Clough construes the sixth commandment as follows: "Thou shalt not kill; but needst not strive/Officiously to keep alive." While not attempting to express the correct balance to be struck in medical practice—the poem satirizes the prevailing hypocrisies of his time— this saying captures the complete independence of not killing from doing everything to keep alive. That is, a physician's rejection of killing does not require him to do everything to keep his patient alive.

To see this while also addressing the issue of causing a patient's death found in terminal sedation, consider what the Hippocratic prohibition rejects. Recall the juror's words: "I will neither give a deadly drug to anyone, though having been asked, nor will I lead the way to such counsel." To give a deadly drug is to give a drug insofar as it is deadly. That is, to give it in order to kill. Here, we speak of the agent's intent, purpose, or what he does deliberately, as a means to an end. One who rejects the giving of a deadly drug insofar as it is deadly rejects having the killing of his patient as either a means to a further goal (to end his patient's pain) or as a goal in itself. For one cannot choose to give a patient a lethal drug insofar as it is lethal without having the death of one's patient as one's means or end. By contrast, one who forgoes the use of a medical intervention or removes the same when doing so results in the patient's death can do so without being intent upon the patient's death. Rather, one (in company, of course, with the patient and/or family) concludes that the medical intervention will not serve (in the case of forgoing its use) or no longer serves (in the case of withdrawing its use) the welfare of the patient. By choosing not at all or no longer to employ the intervention, one need not thereby seek to insure the death of one's patient. Accordingly, one may consistently abjure the giving of a deadly drug to one's patient while not endorsing the employment of every means available to prolong the life of one's patient.

Similarly, if, as is the case in terminal sedation, one cannot adequately treat turmoil due to refractory agonal pain without recourse to a drug that concomitantly depresses or suppresses respiration and causes the terminally ill patient's death, then one may give the drug without thereby being intent upon killing the patient. For one gives the drug insofar as it is palliative, not insofar as it is deadly. Absent a pain-relieving drug or sedative as effective as the one that is also deadly, one lacks a viable alternative to lessen the patient's restlessness in the face of otherwise excruciating pain. Given the inextricability of relieving the patient's distress from concomitantly causing the patient's death, the obligation a physician has so to relieve such discomfort, the imminence of death regardless of what one does, and the consent of the patient or relevant other, a physician reasonably administers the drug.[13] Moreover, one does so without violating the *Oath's* prohibition. For, again, that prohibition bears on the deliberate killing of one's patient. Notably, legal systems prohibiting physicians from euthanizing or assisting in the suicide of one's patient accept terminal sedation as not necessarily incorporating the intent of the patient's death (as do the rejected practices).[14]

3.6 IS THE PROBLEM OF IATROGENIC HARM MOST BASIC?

I have argued that the *Oath's* answer to the problem of iatrogenic harm—particularly as that quandary in its most profound form would conflate the role of healer with that of wounder—founds medical practice as caregiving that especially excludes the egregious injury of killing one's patient (even if done at her request). The physician-philosopher Galen (circa A.D. 129–210) of the Ancient Greek city Pergamon (present-day Bergama, Turkey) tells us in his commentary (one of the fifteen he wrote on the putative works of Hippocrates) concerning the celebrated text from the *Epidemics* "as to diseases, practice two: help or at least, do no harm" (*Epidemics*, 1, 11) that he initially found the advice not to harm one's patient beneath its author. He writes:

> For those who learn the art, I know that, as it was for me, the
> maxim 'be useful or do no harm' seems not to be worthy to
> have been written by Hippocrates; but for those who subse-
> quently practice medicine, I know very well that the force of
> the phrase will be clear. (Jouanna 2012, 264)

Although in the light of experience he revises his opinion of the pri-
macy of avoiding harm to one's patient, Galen's initial response merits
consideration. Does iatrogenic harm—especially role-conflation, noted
in 1.2—constitute the problem the answer to which fundamentally
orients medicine toward caring and away from injuring? Are the pursuit of caring and the avoidance of injury to one's patient in fact primary in medical practice?

Let us consider a salient alternative. Namely, that the central
ethical problem confronting medicine concerns a conflict of interest between the physician's own good and the patient's, or between
egoism and altruism. Before doing so, consider the very terms "ego"
meaning "I" and "alter" meaning "other" from which we derive "egoism" and "altruism." Our current usage dates to about 1830. It traces
back to the sociologist August Comte (1798–1857). One finds the
roots of these two words, respectively, in ancient Greek and classical
Latin. However, the putative conflict between the good of the self
(egoism) and the good of another (altruism)—which seems so obvious to us who habitually consider ourselves atomistic individuals—
does not have the same immediacy for the ancient Greeks or classical
Romans. For they tend to see the good of any one as, at least, not

opposed to the good of others. Moreover, they characteristically regard one's good as congruent with others'. As Aristotle puts it in the *Politics*, man is by nature a political animal, like a bee or an ant, not conceivable as having a meaningful life separate from the polis (Aristotle 1941, 1253a2, 1129). Notably, English instances an atypical language in which the pronoun for the first person singular ("I") requires capitalization, indicating importance. Does this not suggest an overemphasis upon the individual? Perhaps anglophones (among others influenced by modernity) too readily see a duel between the self and others? Nonetheless, let us consider the claim as it bears on medicine.

At the beginning of Plato's *Republic*, Socrates argues about the nature of justice with Thrasymachus—literally, the "rash fighter." Socrates (whose name means "sound strength") maintains that justice benefits all, especially the just. Conversely, Thrasymachus holds that justice is "nothing else than the advantage of the stronger" (Plato 1961, 338c1–2, 588). Exemplifying his name, Thrasymachus recklessly enters and abruptly leaves the discussion concerning justice. Our present interest bears not so much upon their disagreement about justice, but, rather, on what Socrates and Thrasymachus agree upon—at least for a time—concerning the purpose of medicine. Here follows a portion of their discussion:

[SOCRATES:] But tell me, your physician in the precise sense, of whom you were just now speaking, is he a money-maker, an earner of fees, or a healer of the sick? And remember to speak of the physician who is really such.

[THRASYMACHUS:] A healer of the sick. . .

[SOCRATES:] And what of the pilot—the pilot rightly so called—is he a ruler of sailors or a sailor?

[THRASYMACHUS:] A ruler of sailors. (Plato 1961, 341c4-c11, 591)

In their use of the phrases "in the precise sense" and "rightly so called," Socrates and Thrasymachus hope to screen off practitioners of a skill who err in their practice. That is, the physician as a physician, or, in other words, to the extent to which she possesses the medical skill or art, heals the sick. Certainly, an individual physician may inadvertently sicken her patient, but when she does so, she does so insofar as she lacks the medical art, not to the extent to which she possesses it. The same, of course, holds for the captain and other practitioners of an art or skill (using those words interchangeably). In short, the skilled practitioner insofar as he is skilled, acts skillfully and, thereby, achieves his skill's purpose. This clarification naturally leads to an allied question; namely, what is the purpose of a skill? More to the point: is the principal purpose of a skill to secure the well-being of the one who possesses the skill or the good of another?

In answer to this question, slightly further along in the *Republic*, we find:

[SOCRATES:] Then medicine, said I, does not consider the advantage of medicine but of the body?

[THRASYMACHUS:] Yes.

[Socrates:] Nor horsemanship of horsemanship but of horses, nor
does any other art look out for itself—for it has no need—but for
that of which it is the art. (Plato 1961, 342c1-6, 592)

Against Thrasymachus' assertion that justice reduces to what benefits
those in power, Socrates maintains the point that rulers, schoolmasters,
ship-captains, physicians, and horsemen seek not their own advantage, but that of, respectively, the ruled, taught, captained, healed, and
saddled, or the good of citizens, students, sailors, patients, and horses.
According to Socrates, this is so because:

there is no defect or error at all that dwells in any art. Nor
does it befit an art to seek the advantage of anything else than
that of its object. (Plato 1961, 342b2-4, 592)

Socrates tells us that Thrasymachus "assented reluctantly" (Plato 1961,
342e4, 592).

What import does this passage have for our purposes? Given the
tension Socrates notes between the good of the physician and the
good of the patient, one might understandably think that here we
see Socrates identifying the basic ethical issue confronting medicine.
Namely, the fundamental moral issue for a physician will be whether
he puts his good before the good of his patient or subordinates his
welfare to that of his patient's. In short, conflicts of interest: doctor's
versus patient's. This account is not erroneous; rather, it is superficial.
That is, it is true, just not a profound truth the recognition of which
yields much. Before arguing against the view that conflicts of interest

constitute the core of medico-ethical conflicts, however, let us consider the merits of this position.

First, we have Socrates' claim itself. Certainly, Socrates asserts that the physician ought to care for the patient and that this, at least implicitly, can conflict with the physician caring for himself. Second, there is the inherent plausibility of the position, given our tendency to see conflict between the good of one individual and the good of another as almost our natural plight or if not natural, a chronic modern condition. Recall the comment of Thomas Hobbes (a principal modern thinker) that we contrive government to overcome our natural state of a war in which "every man is enemy to every man" that famously renders our lives "solitary, poor, nasty, brutish, and short" (Hobbes 1998, xiii.9, 84). Third, we have a lot of evidence from the history of medicine and of medical ethics that many of the ethical challenges medicine historically and to this day confronts concern this conflict. Indeed, Albert Jonsen, a grey eminence in the history of medical ethics, in a slender rewarding volume holds that "medicine— as an institution, as a practice, as a profession—is dominated by the paradox [of altruism versus self-interest] in its starkest terms" (Jonsen 1990, 6). He says:

> the opposition [between altruism and self-interest] is built into the very structure of medical care and woven into the very fabric of physician's lives. The particular moral problems encountered in medicine are symptoms of this paradox. Many of the psychological troubles of physicians (and their

> families) are fomented by their inability to manage the pres-
> sures it generates. (Jonsen 1990, 5)

Jonsen mentions the various forms that this conflict takes in our time, such as avoiding the provision of unnecessary medical treatments or tests versus financial gain from referral to a facility in which one invests and forgoing futile treatment as without benefit to the patient versus a physician's valued reputation as one who cures (Jonsen 1990, 14–5). Certainly, these and allied examples (such as treating contagious patients from whom one might contract disease) indicate the extent to which acting on behalf of one's patients can conflict with acting on one's own behalf. Nonetheless, this conundrum does not definitively afflict medical practice (as does iatrogenic harm, especially role-conflation).

Consider. While the opposition between altruism and self-interest certainly attends the practice of medicine, it does not do so uniquely or even especially profoundly. Indeed, Jonsen admits that one finds such conflict elsewhere, just not as ubiquitously as in medicine. That is, this is not the vexing ethical problem the solution to which inaugurates medicine as a profession. It is, rather, the precise difficulty noted by Socrates which confronts anyone occupying a role charged with the welfare of another. We call such roles "fiduciary," from the Latin *fides*, meaning "faith" or "trust."

In fiduciary or trust-based relationships, such as teacher-student, doctor- or nurse-patient, lawyer- or accountant-client, or religious leader-congregant, we have the one who trusts (the trustor) and the one trusted (the trustee). Conflicts of interest plague fiduciary relationships. Indeed, because they do so with such predictability, fiduciary relationships often require the avoidance, not only of conflicts of interest, but even the *appearance* of a conflict of interest. For example, when certifying a company's statements of profit and loss, certified public accountants must assure the public not only that they do not have a real conflict of interest, by, say, directly owning shares in the company; they must also not even appear to be subject to such a conflict, by, for example, having a spouse, child, or close relative employed by that company.

We can make comparable points relying on the notion of a caretaker. In any caretaking role, one acts on behalf of another's welfare. Indeed, this constitutes Socrates' general point: numerous roles share the feature of one taking care of another. All such arts (he uses the Greek term *technē*) charge the artists with the welfare of the one (person, being, or thing) cared for, not that of the caregiver. Indeed, one common complaint of caregivers as diverse as veterinarians, physicians, lawyers, accountants, and professors goes as follows: "In ___ school, they taught me how to care for ___, not the business, professional development, self-interested side of ___." Of course, successful practitioners must discern how to keep body and soul together in part in order to keep practicing their relevant art. This, however, as Socrates notes, does not constitute part of the art. The care of the relevant subject (or object) makes up the entirety of the art. Care of the art and of the artist serve as adjuvant arts. Proverbially, one notes how artisans fail to furnish themselves with the very good they provide to others: "The estate lawyer dies intestate." The attorney lacks what he diligently prepares for others.

In short, conflicts of interest attend fiduciary and caretaking roles. Insofar as medicine instances such a role, conflicts of interest attend medicine. They do not, however, do so uniquely. Rather, the predicament of iatrogenic harm—especially as instanced in the conflation of injuring with healing—singularly afflicts medicine. Moreover, the *Oath's* response to this dilemma does in fact define medicine as we know it.

3.7 FORSWEARING OTHER INJURIES AND INJUSTICES: SEXUAL RELATIONS AND GOSSIP

As we conclude this chapter acknowledging that the vexing issue confronting medical practice concerns the caregiver adopting the role of wounder, a final question arises. Namely, has Hippocrates correctly identified the injuries to be avoided in the care of one who labors under illness? Put in slightly different terms, does the *Oath* discern the most worrisome vulnerabilities of the sick? Of course, put this way, one notes that "vulnerable" itself means "subject to being wounded, hurt, injured, maimed," from the previously noted Latin *vulnus* for "wound." Certainly, vulnerability characterizes the sick, subject at the very least to the wounds necessary to the work of healing them (what I refer to in 1.2 as wounds of treatment or therapy) and, more worrisomely, to deliberate injury. While not proposed as an exhaustive list of harms, does the *Oath* neglect injuries meriting inclusion among the list of killing, sexually exploiting, and gossiping? Moreover, what of contemporary concerns, such as respect for the patient as autonomous and the associated need for complete truth-telling?

Given its salience in the *Oath*, which reflects its import for mortals, I have dwelt at length on the grounds for a physician's forswearing patient-killing. As noted in 2.2.3, the *Oath* specifically mentions two other injuries and injustices, namely sexual misconduct and spreading news abroad, gossiping, or what we might now refer to as violating patient confidentiality. Do these merit specification? If so, why? Recall the relevant passage:

> Into as many houses as I enter, I will go into in order to benefit the sick, being free from all voluntary injustice and corruption, especially sexual acts with the bodies of females and of males, of free and of slaves. About whatever in therapy I see or hear, or also outside of therapy concerning the life of men, that ought never to be spoken out, I will be silent, holding such things not to be spoken.

As mentioned in 2.2.3, the juror swears to avoid these injustices in the context of crossing the household's threshold. Accordingly, the physician forswears these acts partially insofar as he has been granted the privilege of entering the house, something reserved to trusted non-family members. In this respect, one might think of these promises as bearing on the physician, not so much as physician, but rather as one entering the household. We would err, however, were we to think that the juror does not speak more precisely in his role as physician, as we will see shortly.

The sweeping, categorical, unqualified character of the *Oath* on these matters strikes one: "of females and of males, of free and of slaves" and "whatever in therapy I see or hear, or also outside of therapy." The juror leaves no wiggle room, as it were. Of course, the juror does not enumerate (nor could one, given the countless number of ways one can stray from the right path) all of the voluntary injustices and corruptions that one might perpetrate. He does, however, single out these two of sexual exploitation and the violation of an encompassing confidentiality inclusive of patient, family, and household.

Consider forswearing sexual relations. In order to practice medicine well, one needs the patient to remove his or her clothes so that one may examine the subject. Such medical requests must be emphatically distinguished from sexual conduct. Moreover, while we humans naturally find one another sexually attractive, the Greek context merits remark. As male, a physician would be assumed potentially to have sexual interest in members of the household in accordance with the very words of the *Oath*: females, males, free or slave. In addition to distinguishing the sometimes necessary request for disrobement from an aphrodisiacal act, the juror has to address and deny the applicability of this presumption.

With respect to confidentiality, the juror forswears gossiping about what arises "in therapy or apart from therapy." Medical practice gives rise to knowledge about intimate matters concerning the patient and the wider household that ought never (in the words of the juror) to be spoken about abroad. Of course, to discern what ought never to be spoken about abroad requires judgment. As subject to judgment, it admits of disagreement. Whatever the case, the physician here promises the patient, family, and household to exercise discretion while recognizing the category of what ought never to be spoken about abroad. With these promises in place, the physician can be trusted to cross over the threshold without guile, for the benefit of the sick. Yet what of other injuries, such as inadequate respect for patient autonomy or less than complete truth-telling?

The injuries the *Oath* explicitly mentions have an ageless character such that they always confront one offering therapy. The human condition being what it is—generally messy in its mortality, sexuality, and curiosity—sick humans will want to be killed by their physicians (and others will want the sick to be killed); patients (among others) and physicians will find one another sexually attractive; and everyone will be interested in what the physician knows about the patients' mortality, sexuality, and allied details. That is, the prohibitions against killing, sexual relations with patients (and others encountered in therapy), and gossiping have the salience the *Oath* indicates. By contrast, respecting a patient's autonomy and telling the whole unvarnished truth have less to do with the human way of being and more to do with a certain time and place in which we humans conceive of ourselves as individual atomistic beings and in which doctors presumably have more to tell patients. Of course, the point here does not consist in a dismissal of the import of patient autonomy or truth-telling (or to suggest that the Hippocratic physician does not tell the truth and respect a patient's autonomy). Rather, one hopes properly to locate their significance as of greater relevance to our time and our place in contrast to a larger set of times and places. In this respect, the *Oath* presents a perennial ethic for the practice of the medical profession. Hence, it addresses the most prominent offenses. This observation brings us to our final chapter, the *Oath* vis-à-vis medicine as a profession. To that consideration I now turn.

Chapter 4
OATH, PROFESSION, AND AUTONOMY

T hus far we have considered the Hippocratic *Oath* in its specifics. Yet (for the moment putting to the side what one promises), why have a medical oath at all? Why vow?[1] Why profess? Numerous reasons bear remark; some implicate medicine as a profession—that is, as a doing in which practitioners openly impose norms on themselves, an autonomous praxis as will be established in what follows. Thus, in this final chapter I investigate the connections between a medical promise, a medical profession, and medical autonomy. I conclude by noting that the enduring legacy of the *Oath* consists in the conception and establishment of doctoring as a profession, a practice incorporating its own publicly avowed ethic.

4.1 OATH AND PROFESSION

Among the oldest extant references to the *Oath*, we find that of Scribonius Largus, an early first century (A.D. circa 14–54) physician who practiced medicine in Rome. In *Compositiones*—Latin for "pre-scriptions," his only surviving work, in which he presents some 271 pharmacological recipes ranging from tooth-cleaning medicaments to drugs for treating snakebite—he writes:

> Hippocrates, the founder of our profession, handed on to our discipline an oath by which it is sworn that no physician will either give or demonstrate to pregnant women any drug abort-ing a conceived child. Thus he greatly prepared the minds of his disciples for humanity. For how much more abominable will those men judge it to do harm to a fully formed human being who consider it wicked to injure the uncertain hope of an unborn child? Therefore, the conservation of the name and honor of medicine with a holy and devoted heart has been greatly valued by every man who has behaved himself according to Hippocrates' credo: "For medicine is the science of healing, not of harming." (Hamilton 1986, 214)[2]

Here we encounter the connection of present interest (putting to the side the ascription of the *Oath* to Hippocrates—I do not produce Scribonius as a witness for that claim). Namely, that between medicine as a profession and medicine as involving an oath. How do the two relate?

Scribonius refers to Hippocrates as the "founder of our profes-sion"—in the original Latin "*conditor nostrae professionis*" (Largus 1983, 2). [3] As one medical historian notes concerning Scribonius' use of *pro-fessio*, the term specifically implicates an ethical commitment:

> This word [*professio*], in the language of his [Scribonius'] time, was applied to workmanship in preference to the older and morally indefinite terms, in order to emphasize the ethical connotations of work, the idea of an obligation or a duty on the part of those engaged in the arts and crafts. (Edelstein 1967, 339)

The profession of medicine as involving unique ethical commitments and the *Oath*, for example, as public declaration mutually implicate one another. Indeed, so much so that one reasonably regards the taking of the oath-proper as transformative of the—to use Edelstein's words—"older and morally indefinite" underlying technique into a profession. That is, in keeping with Scribonius' usage, a practice incorporating role-defining ethical commitments.

Etymologically, "profession" captures the oath-taking aspect of such a practice. "Pro-" means "in front of" or "openly;" "-fession" comes from the Latin *fateri*, which means "to declare." Thus, by definition, a professional makes a public declaration. Minimally, that might amount simply to saying "I am a ___." Indeed, an archaic Roman usage of *professio* refers to the statement one makes before tax authorities concerning one's occupation. By extension, it names one's calling, applying particularly to vocations that involve norms of craft-conduct (as Scribonius' usage attests). Practitioners who deal with adequately weighty matters profess to uphold their craft's standards. Accordingly, among the first uses of *professio* one finds medicine—so described by the layman Aulus Cornelius Celsus (circa 25 B.C.— A.D. 50) in the preface to his work *De Medicina* (*Concerning Medicine*).[4]

Solemnly declaring before others that for which one stands characterizes a profession. We regard medicine as a paradigmatic profession. Accordingly, given the intimate connection between openly declaring what one stands for and membership in a profession, physicians take an oath. This rationale, however, might appear entirely nominal, as if referring to the healing art as a profession alone grounds the taking of an iatric vow. Such an account touches merely the surface. Reflection on the connections between swearing an oath and the healer's practice reveals deeper reasons.

4.2 FURTHER REASONS FOR A MEDICAL OATH

By marriage vows spouses promise fidelity. By oaths of office, elected officials, judges, lawyers, and police swear to act on behalf of the common goods entrusted to them. By religious vows, nuns and sisters promise celibacy, poverty, and obedience.[5] As these examples indicate, the practice of public promising attends particularly serious roles. Matrimonial vows address one's spousal station. Political oaths pertain to offices devoted to upholding the laws of the land. Religious vows bear on vocations concerning God. Sex, justice, and divinity instance significant matters. Therefore, posts concerning such affairs themselves have import, as professing indicates.

The above suggests the first reason I will note (of seven) for taking a medical oath. Namely, that medicine concerns vital affairs, as do the other fora within which we characteristically find oath-taking: marriage, bearing on sexual relations; law, on justice; and religion, on divinity. Specifically, medicine addresses our susceptibility to illness, decline, and death and our associated need for therapy. Caring for humans as beings subject to wounds—vulnerable—constitutes a weighty doing; medicine has the gravity necessary for the solemn practice of oath-taking. Hence, physicians fittingly take oaths. By contrast, one might find it something of a stretch (bordering on the humorous) were hairstylists or cosmeticians, for example, to take solemn vows. For the goods at issue in grooming lack the import requisite for the taking of an oath.

Second, the taking of a public oath emphasizes the deliberate nature of what one does. It indicates reflective commitment or devotion: literally, the taking of a vow (from the Latin, *de-vovere*: to dedicate, or solemnly promise one's self by a vow—*votum*). As the first reason indicates, an oath concerns significant matters. This second point suggests that, additionally, it instances gravitas regarding those affairs. According to the first point, one does not take an oath concerning the frivolous. In keeping with the second, one does not take an oath frivolously. Rather, the taking of an oath itself suggests one has extensively thought about what one promises; one knowledgeably and willingly promises.

This brings me to the third reason for making a public promise; namely, to help insure that one will, in fact, keep the promise. This puzzles. If one deliberately commits oneself to some goal, why think that doing so in speech before others will assist one in realizing that goal? Students of promising note that it facilitates the realization of that which one promises. At least three motives appear operative in the keeping of our profession (if I may so use the term). First, when we publicly promise we regard ourselves as committed to that to which we promise. We see our own act as deliberate, serious, and as involving a high level of commitment. This, in turn, moves us to be true to our own promise (for its own sake, as it were.) Second, we make such a promise to and before others. Moreover, others so understand us to have promised. We thereby create in others expectations that we, in turn, wish to fulfill.[6] Third, because a solemn public promise characteristically involves invoking God—or, formulaically, "all that I hold sacred"—we keep our promise in part because we call as witness the being (or reality) that we regard as of greatest import and transcendence. Notably, one cannot readily deceive such a witness. Thus, professing facilitates by various mechanisms (probably not and perhaps never to be comprehensively understood) our very keeping—our making true—of that which we promise.

Fourth, an oath focuses subsequent deliberation. For it determines that about which the one who takes it will and will not deliberate. A spouse deliberates about how to express love to wife or husband while not deliberating about whether to have sexual relations with someone else. Similarly, when problems of sickness or poverty (or wealth) arise, the wedding vows direct the spouse to deliberate about how to honor the promise. By its general determination of the spouse toward certain goods and away from others, it focuses the spouse's agency on what to think about. This benefits her. For it answers one of the chief questions she confronts as she enters into deliberation; namely, what should I think about? What problems require solution? By eliminating salient distractions and directing her toward the good to be pursued, an oath facilitates the juror's effective deliberation (and, thereby, further serves her keeping of the promise).

Fifth, by delimiting the field of activity well, an oath facilitates the advancement of the practice. Just as the rules of a sport in part determine what constitutes athletic excellence in it, so too, the norms to which one commits in a professional oath partially further that practice's development. Consider, for example, the art of rhetoric (discounting the pejorative connotation that often attends the term). Imagine an oath taken by rhetoricians. Suppose, further, and in keeping with the classical conception, that the rhetorician swears to persuade his audience to hold reasonable positions by means of cogent arguments while forswearing to convince his audience by falsehoods. As those who engage in public debate acknowledge, lying, fabricating, and fudging chronically tempt one to employ them with a view to convincing one's audience. Of course, public debate can have a warlike, agonistic character. Proverbially, truth is the first casualty of war. The rhetorician, however, does not employ falsehood, as his profession rules it out of bounds. Accordingly, he must convince his audience relying on alternative resources—humorous stories, apt examples, poignant narratives, eloquent phrases—that he must discover within the boundaries he acknowledges. Thereby, he advances and excels—as all advancement and excellence occurs—within limits. Of course, to excel is to run out ahead of others. One can do so only on a defined, limited, bounded course. For absent the way being restricted, there is no ahead of, and, thereby, no excelling. Were he to recur to lying, he would to that extent preclude the development of the art and of his own artistry. Perhaps in this instance he would not discover the efficacy of or his capacity for humor. By his very choice not to lie, he, of course, renders the accomplishment of his task more difficult. Absent so constraining himself, however, he would not have a discernible task. For the paths leading to the accomplishment of his goal partially depend upon that very restriction in order to be defined. Moreover, as noted, to determine what it would be for him to excel, he (and others) must delimit the way on which he could run ahead by ruling in and out certain means of persuasion. Paradoxically, this self-binding by oath also leads him toward perfection of his art and discovery of his field of activity. What resources are within bounds that, were he to have recurred to lying, he would not have seen? Consider: how many lies are told simply because of unwarranted fear, easily remedied ignorance, or lack of imagination?

As the original Greek word for oath (*horkos*) indicates in its relation to the word for fence (*herkos*, as noted in 2.2), a professional vow delimits the boundaries within which one will practice one's art. It defines the practice in term of ends which and means by which one will (or will not) seek. Thereby, it helps determine, identify, and foster excellence within that practice.

Sixth, an oath always explains and can also justify one's conduct. A promise serves as both a reason to do something (and, thus, an explanation for one's doing it) and, other things being equal, a justification for doing it.[7] Consider the marriage vow. Were someone to suggest adultery, a spouse could explain and justify not so acting by referring to the matrimonial promise. The vow explains the rebuff. Moreover, in light of the pledge's rightness, it justifies one's rejection of extramarital relations. Hence, "I am married" both explains and justifies one's refusal of infidelity.

Implicit in and following upon the above points comes an encompassing, seventh, and final reason for the taking of a medical oath; namely, to realize professional medical autonomy. "Autonomy" derives from the Greek *autos* meaning "self" and *nomos* meaning "law." Ancient Greeks of the fifth and fourth centuries b.c. (e.g., Thucydides and Demosthenes) use *autonomos* to refer primarily to citizens living under their own laws. By extension they use it to encompass an individual acting under his own judgment (e.g., Sophocles so employs it).[8] By a medical oath, the professing impose a medical law, custom, or ethic upon themselves. Accordingly, we aptly speak of medical professionals as autonomous.

By solemnly swearing medical practitioners inaugurate medicine as an autonomous practice having its own norms. An apt oath founds, defines, communicates, and (thereby) protects a practice's standards before, to, and from practitioners, prospective students, patients, political authorities, and the public. Healers establish and enunciate their professional relationship with others by publicly declaring the goods on behalf of which and the limits within which they will practice medicine. A medical vow limns and promulgates physicians' commitments. The mender's pledge educates a wide audience about the most salient therapeutic benefits and boundaries. Made aware of the profession's character by the solemn promise, patients know that to which physicians devote themselves, as do students who want to learn the art so understood. Similarly, those in authority can understand and appropriately relate to the practice. Moreover, the avowal enables the general public to identify and have due recourse to the profession's members.

Absent such a declaration, physicians jeopardize their ability to determine what is and what is not medicine and, thereby, what they will and will not do. By taking an oath, they safeguard their practice from the inevitable attempts to employ medicine (a powerful technique) for purposes not in keeping with its commitments. Moreover, this declaration disciplines members who might otherwise abuse the relevant skills. Hence, by a solemn medical pledge, doctors inoculate themselves against subornation to the service of other ends, some of which may prove alien, indeed, even opposed to the goods sought by the medical profession. In short, an oath instances, defines, transmits, represents, sustains, and furthers the medical profession's autonomy.

The above considerations indicate salient reasons for having a medical oath. The final reason noted—the realization of autonomy by means of professing—now leads us to reflect on professional autonomy.

4.3 PROFESSIONAL AUTONOMY

A profession possesses an autonomy independent from what law and society forbid and allow to others. Hence, professionals can do or must not do acts that others cannot do or may do.

Society acknowledges professional autonomy because it serves the common good, society's project. A civil engineer enjoys right of passage over land while being obligated to report unsanitary conditions.

He does so because his actions further civil order, health, and safety. A certified public accountant retains a right of client confidentiality while being required to avoid the perception of a conflict of interest, for her work advances commerce, the cement of society. A surgeon may cut into a patient but must not betray the patient's confidence, for a citizen's health sometimes depends on the commission of what would otherwise be assault. Needless to say, a layman may not trespass, certify, nor incise, while he need not report dangers, appear unbiased, nor keep a secret. The autonomy of a profession amounts to a privilege enjoyed by and reserved to practitioners. As "privilege" suggests, it is a unique, private (from the Latin *privus*) norm or law (*lex*), an ethic internal to a practice. What does it mean to speak of a norm as intrinsic to a profession?

Briefly, a professional practice has goods native to itself the pursuit of which define that activity. The preservation or restoration of and attention to a patient's health instance the goods definitive of medical practice. The civil goods of public health, safety, and order attributable to sanitary sewage, clean drinking water, proper drainage of storm run-off, and overall good design of municipal infrastructure amount to the goods specifying civil engineering. The list of goods indigenous to professional practices could go on to include the goods tended to by soldiers, captains, judges, teachers, architects, nurses, police, accountants, pilots, actuaries, and professors, among others. Such goods differ from external goods such as wealth, honor, power, and fame. For these latter goods—and emphatically, they are goods—attend all practices while belonging to none. One can inherit wealth, win the lottery, or come by it through virtuosity in a professional practice. External goods are good, are important in sustaining professionals (and, thereby, professions), but neither belong to nor define a specific practice nor practices more generally.

The inherent ethic of a professional practice concerns the practitioner's care for the internal goods—that is, the goods definitive of that professional practice.[9] The interior ethic may at times repeat more general ethical norms, such as "do not lie," but it does so in its own voice, with a view focused upon the goods entrusted to it. More importantly, the constitutional ethic does not merely echo broader moral commitments. Rather, at its center it addresses the goods entrusted to the practice and the threats confronting those goods. As argued thus far, professing amounts to stating the goods on behalf of which one stands while, as necessary, forswearing what opposes those goods. Having sketched the outlines of an ethic internal to a practice, let us return to our principal concern, medicine's autonomy.

Medical professing implicates medical autonomy, which, in turn, entails a medical law, ethic, or custom. Concerning the medical custom, a number of questions arise. First, as law, what characteristics would such an ethic have? Second, what would the medical code mandate in its most generic least controvertible form (albeit controverted as it becomes specified, as we will see in 4.4)? Third and finally, what do professed internal caregiving norms ask of physicians and others? Having considered why medicine aptly involves professing, let us address these salient affiliated questions.

4.3.1 Professional Autonomy: The Internal Therapeutic Ethic as Law

First, consider the most general features of any plausible ethic (a word of Greek derivation originally meaning "custom") physicians might lay down for themselves in the form of a medical custom or law—for example, the oath-proper's *nomos iētrikos*. "Law," of course, references a vast territory. The Dominican friar Thomas Aquinas (circa A.D. 1224–1274), the great light of the Middle Ages, offers a succinct yet encompassing definition: "promulgated rational rule ordered to the common good made by those who have care of the community."[10] Hence, Thomas proposes that law has four features: promulgated, rational measure, communally ordered, and authoritatively fashioned. He understands law analogously. That is, across diverse fora—the primary being actual legislatures—laws retain these core elements in a parallel, not identical manner. As it proves fruitful, I follow his lead.

One readily discerns how these four features relate to medical promising. First, by an oath physicians publicly declare their norms (as noted in 4.2). Second, a medical vow must have reason on its side, instancing rational rules in contrast to the arbitrary, willful, or capricious. Third, it does so if the goods shared among practitioners and patients ground the reasons offered on behalf of the adopted norms, in contrast to private goods the enjoyment of which necessarily exclude others (and, hence, are private).[11] Among the more prominent common medical goods, one finds the health of patients entrusted to and cared for by physicians, the practice-preserving medical education of novices, and the advancement of medical knowledge and technique—all for the benefit of the sick. If there are salient harms to be avoided in attending to the ill, preserving the practice, or advancing the same, they will also figure in the medical law. Fourth, practitioners trusted by and in the company of patients discern the therapeutic goods to be pursued and bads to be avoided. In light of these experiential insights and the authority they confer, healers will develop customs and fashion general codes for caregiving, medical laws as it were. In summation, by professing physicians promulgate reasonable measures to further communal medical goods authoritatively discovered. As noted, two further questions remain. First, what more specifically might the most basic least dubitable norm internal to medicine enjoin? Second, what does the self-government of the profession require of its members and others such as patients and political authorities? Let us answer these questions.

4.3.2 Professional Autonomy: The Basic Internal Medical Norm

To address the first question, one must attend to medicine as manifesting practical reason. Aquinas (following Aristotle, to whom he refers with the honorific "the Philosopher") notes that reason operates in two modes: speculatively (theoretically)—when we know something about reality—and practically—when by acting we make something real. We have one faculty, reason, that we employ diversely either to apprehend the world (know it) or to affect it (cause it to be this way or that).[12]

Thomas notes that in both instances we possess first principles, the axioms in accordance with which reason theorizes or practices.

The first precept of reason employed speculatively approximates to what we might more commonly speak of as the "principle of non-contradiction." That is, a thing cannot be x and not-x (at the same time and in the same respect). More succinctly, as a logician might write it: ~ (p · ~p). Again, in other words, "not (p and not-p)." No matter how one puts it, hardly a subject of debate. Indeed, Aristotle, the father of systematic logic, considers the maxim so basic that we cannot subject it to debate. For we rely on it in both all we assert and all we deny.

In the arena of reason employed practically, Aquinas proposes a comparably fundamental tenet. Since it governs conduct, he refers to it as a law. Since it is basic, he considers it a primary law, from which all practical measures derive. It commands: "the good is to be done and pursued; and, the bad is to-be-avoided."[13] Again, no controversy to be found here, although, since it is a prescriptive law, we can, of course, break it.[14] This rule, Thomas proposes, amounts to the first ethical insight—which one cannot fail to have. The intuitive obviousness of that *principium* interests Aquinas, for it suggests a shared innate standard for judging our conduct. Of course (as will be addressed shortly in 4.4), one—as does the Dominican friar—asks and disputes answers to the question: "what is good; what is bad?" One does so knowing, however, that the good is to-be-done and pursued; the bad, to-be-avoided. What the angelic doctor finds remarkable is this obvious truth. He does not seek to bring the dictum to our attention as if we did not or (even) could not know it. Indeed, were it not evident to us, he would clearly be mistaken about its foundational character. Rather, he proposes that we consider its primal nature. The scholar from Aquino suggests this criterion as first in the entire forum of human activity. In diverse fields of conduct, we encounter specifications of this maxim as practitioners pursue goods and avoid (opposed) bads internal to diverse practices.

In this light, consider the elementary medical axiom: "as to diseases, practice two: help or do not harm"—briefly mentioned in 1.2's discussion of iatrogenic harm.[15] Again, this may be the urtext for the pithy "first, do no harm" or, in Latin, "*primum, non nocere*," whose origins have yet to be adequately determined. As noted in 1.2, the Greek infinitive (*askein*) connotes "practice skillfully." It suggests the development of finesse. Commenting on this advice found in the *Epidemics*, Galen of Pergamon—the second- and early-third-century A.D. philosopher-doctor who rose from physician to gladiators to become court physician to, among others, the Roman Emperor Marcus Aurelius—has much of interest to say:

> I for one thought previously that this maxim was insignificant and that it was not worthy of Hippocrates. Indeed, I thought that everyone understood that the doctor should do the best for his patients, and certainly not harm them. But when I saw reputable doctors quite rightly charged for what they had done whilst performing a phlebotomy, in bathing someone or administering a drug, or wine or cold water, I understood that this may have happened to Hippocrates himself, and that in any case it necessarily happened to many other

doctors in his time; and from that moment, I considered, if by chance I had to administer some powerful drug to a patient, to examine beforehand myself not only how I would be useful in obtaining my aim, but also how I would not harm him. Thus, I have never done anything without beforehand taking care, in case I do not achieve my aim, of not harming the patient in any way. By contrast, some doctors, like those who throw a dice, tend to administer remedies to patients which, if they do not work, cause them great damage. For those who learn the art, I know that, as it was for me, the maxim 'be useful or do no harm' seems not to be worthy to have been written by Hippocrates; but for those who subsequently practice medicine, I know very well that the force of the phrase will be clear; and if it occurs that after an erroneous use of a strong drug a patient dies, they will understand most clearly the force of what Hippocrates advised. (Jouanna 2012, 264)

Galen recounts his own realization over time of the full import of this pithy dictum. At the beginning of his career, the maxim appeared trivial. He regarded it as beneath Hippocrates' attention, known by all. The onetime physician to gladiators comes to realize, however, that his initial attitude belongs to those "who learn the art," or students. Novices (as did he) erroneously regard this insight as not meriting Hippocrates' remark. Those who "subsequently practice medicine" appreciate the profundity of Hippocrates' saying. "From that moment" when the physician-philosopher first appreciated its import, he has never done anything without observing this practical precept. He aptly notes how basic this norm is. Rudimentary, yet deeply important. Galen's reflection upon Hippocrates' famous aphorism echoes within the field of medicine Aquinas' illuminating discussion of the first practical principle.

This axial medical tenet instances a first practical therapeutic principle around which professional conduct turns. This rule and those that ramify from it amount to the code that medical practitioners follow. One might understandably consider such an axiom relatively contentless, such as Thomas' "pursue and do the good; avoid the bad." While "as to diseases, practice two: help and do not harm" appears gossamer-like, it has more substance than one might first apprehend—as Galen indicates. Let us partially articulate its import as an ethic internal to medicine.

First, it equates to a uniquely medical rule of practice, bearing as it does upon one who suffers from a disease. Hence, it focuses on the goods to be sought (and bads to be avoided) concerning the patient's health, the good definitive of medical therapy, internal to the practice. This may seem beneath notice. However, one discerns its relevance by noting that the sick individual remains subject to other goods and bads. For example, the diseased person also has financial concerns. Such concerns, however, do not figure determinatively in the physician's practicing medicine as do the boons and banes concerning the patient's physical health. A doctor's role-defining responsibility concerns the sick individual's physical, not fiscal, welfare—or, needless to say, her intellectual, political, or social well-being. Organic, physical, psychosomatic goods and bads concern the healer as healer: specifically, uniquely, definitively. This brings us to our second observation concerning the significance of this basic norm.

Of the physician, the law (using that term analogously) demands practice while suggesting the development of finesse, practice making perfect. Following this golden medical rule, the physician and his peers repeatedly act and refrain from acting in certain ways and in certain circumstances, developing standards of care. Always practicing, they constantly refine and revise these ways of acting (and not acting). This indicates the dynamic and progressive aspect of medicine. Practitioners must constantly apply themselves to become adroit, even virtuoso. They do so always mindful of both the fixed end (assisting the sick) and the boundary concerning the pursuit of that end (not harming). Advancing toward this goal on the bounded path, they excel—excellence occurring only within boundaries (as noted in 4.2). By healers' achievements and the sharing of excellence (via peer- and novice-education), the practice develops. A third observation concerning this pithy imperative naturally follows.

Attend, sustain, assist, cure the sick; while doing so, avoid harming. Yet, excellent therapy often necessarily involves hurting—as noted in 1.2 and 3.2. Consider the use of any medicament in the care of the sick. As Paracelsus says: "all things are poison and nothing is not poison, only the dose makes it to be a thing that is not poison."[16] This holds of all regimens (if we may use Hippocrates' all-encompassing term). Ingested, even too much water can prove noxious. Moreover, and more importantly for our present inquiry, properly dosed drugs typically have undesirable side effects. Aspirin—whose active ingredient is a close cousin of salicylic acid, found in willow-tree-root, one of the oldest continuously used drugs in history—in addition to its beneficial anti-inflammatory effects has ineliminable deleterious side effects, such as irritation of the stomach and bowels. Does one abide by the foundational tenet by not giving aspirin because it also has obnoxious effects? No. That amounts to complete therapeutic nihilism, the abdication of caregiving. Given that Hippocrates' maxim does not recommend such a path, how ought we understand it?

Galen's ruminations illustrate the import of this axiom. For he emphasizes deliberation in one's helping and not harming: "I considered," "to examine beforehand," "how I would be useful. . . but also how I would not harm," "I have never done anything without beforehand taking care." Deliberately, purposefully, intentionally help and—given that helping inevitably involves harming as an obnoxious side-effect (cutting, nauseating, etc.) —deliberately reduce harm as much as therapeutically possible while never purposefully, electively, deliberately, or intentionally harming. The golden medical rule definitively orients the therapist toward trying to help while ruling out trying to harm.

To sum up, the first internal medical norm mandates the deliberate, excelling pursuit of patients' health while avoiding all elective harm. Notably, this amounts to a rational measure ordered to the communal good of health arrived at authoritatively via lived practice (as Galen indicates). Were it promulgated by public professing, it would clearly instance a medical law. This brings us to our final question concerning what the internal standard requires of, among others, physicians. Before answering this question, the preceding calls for an observation; namely, that professional medicine cannot amount to a technique exclusively. Allow me to establish this point.

4.3.3 Professional Autonomy: Medicine not Solely a Technique

To see that medicine as a profession cannot amount wholly to a method, let us briefly rehearse our passage to this juncture. We began by noting the intimate connection between vowing and medicine as a profession, the latter of which involves autonomy. Self-lawing, of course, involves a medical law, the general characteristics of which we enunciated. We then presented and elaborated upon the most general least controvertible medical rule. Now we consider the import of this ethic intrinsic to medicine as a profession. Simply put, incorporating an ethic, medicine cannot equate entirely to know-how. A technique, in itself, does not include determination toward an end and away from what opposes that end, while an ethic necessarily does.

Consider. The grammarian as grammarian fashions both the most grammatical and least grammatical sentences. In deliberately making the least grammatical sentence, the grammarian exercises the grammatical art and displays virtuosity in that knack. For grammar consists of knowing how to relate words to one another in sentences. Purposefully doing this badly can illustrate excellent practice just as thoroughly as doing it well. Indeed, the very best at it can do it worse than the less skillful.

Witness Geoffrey Chaucer (if I may focus on him grammatically, borrowing his poetic license, as it were). In his hilariously bad *Sir Thopas*, he puts his expertise fully on display. Only a master such as Chaucer could write a poem to which the Host rightly responds "*Mine eris aken of thy drasty speche!*" (Chaucer 2005, 923, 509). His ability to make such dregs in speech amidst the incomparable *Canterbury Tales* partially explains why we continue to read Chaucer some six centuries past his demise. Even as he versifies badly, he exemplifies verbal facility.

The finesse of the physician, by contrast, does not equate entirely to a method. For it necessarily integrates health as the end of its activities while precluding deliberate, chosen, intended sickening. Hence, medical virtuosity necessarily excludes adroit injuring. As professional, medicine cannot be adequately understood absent acknowledgment of an ethic internal to itself, involving more than know-how. Yet one might object that an oath could consist solely of a promise of technical expertise. If so, could not a medical profession amount entirely to technique?

Consider this demurral. To what would such an oath amount? Something along the lines of, "I vow, as to diseases, to practice (full stop)." Practice what? To heal or to spread diseases? One practices acts. Acts—the means employed to achieve ends—require ends. Thus, practicing requires ends. For by practicing one tries to improve one's way of achieving the relevant goals. Hence, she who promises to practice skillfully without specifying goods (and bads) swears absurdly. Moreover, she would not know what she vows. The import of her own pledge would remain largely opaque to her, to be determined by technical possibility, demand, and legality (presumably). Were she asked to what she has committed herself, she would reply "I do not know; I did solemnly declare to do it well." This amounts to a rash, reckless, heedless oath. One finds no profession here. Thus, a medical profession cannot amount solely to a devotion to technical expertise. (In passing, one notes that one could avow in an Apollonian fashion, discussed in chapter 3, to practice curing and spreading diseases. The insurmountable difficulty confronting this vow concerns how such contradictory ends can be reasonably reconciled in one practice. Such a promise must remain arbitrary, capricious, and unreasonable, an unprincipled profession.) Having shown that professional medical practice does not comport with medicine conceived of as entirely a technique, let us now limn what professional medical autonomy calls for from physicians and others.

4.3.4 Professional Autonomy: Salient Claims

Physicians' regard for their own medical autonomy has three foci: selves, peers, and the wider public—most prominently patients. Of course, first and most importantly, it requires a doctor to keep her own promise vis-à-vis the precept and the norms deriving from it. Second, each having disciplined herself, she and her peers must govern one another, regulating each other's practices. They do so (in private and public) by, among other means, emulation and corrective critique, praise and blame, referral and non-referral, and licensing and its revocation. Third, having duly ruled themselves and peers, physicians must articulate the autonomy of the profession to patients, the public, and political authorities. To do so, doctors must educate those outside the profession concerning their medical commitments. This becomes particularly incumbent on healers when the sick, the putatively ill, or others (such as the state officials of North Carolina—noted in 3.3.3—who sought physician-participation in capital punishment) seek to use medicine in manners not in keeping with its internal ethic.

Some think that the conjunction of technical feasibility, legality, and a competent individual's desire for a physician's assistance tend to obligate a doctor to supply the relevant demanded intervention, regardless of her profession. They find this supposed duty even more pronounced insofar as the law allows only physicians to perform certain acts. According to such thinkers, mere fiat transforms politicians, legislators, and voters into physicians—bringing to mind the adage "if 'ifs' and 'ands' were pots and pans, there'd be no need for tinkers' hands." Indeed, no need for menders', either. Such thinkers entirely eradicate professionalism from medicine.

As the foregoing has duly established, however, medical professing incorporates an internal ethic. Absent compatibility with a professed ethic, those who want to use medical technique to achieve some desideratum do not thereby have a just claim on physicians' collaboration. Lacking congruence with a medical profession, if some regard the use of medical know-how as so exigent, lawmakers can allow competent others with different principles to meet the perceived need, as surely as demand creates supply. Presumably, this would serve medical autonomy. If so, such measures could count one argument in their favor.

In a context of contested claims to the physician's capabilities, contemporary liberal society acknowledges medical autonomy by respecting professional conscience. It does so most pointedly by honoring professional conscientious objection when parties' claims conflict. Let us briefly consider this eventuality.

"Conscience" comes from the Latin *con-* meaning "really" (or "with") and *scire* meaning "to know." As we use it exclusively to refer to moral knowledge, the word suggests that our conscience concerns what we really know to be good or bad, the ethical commitments of which we are certain. Moreover, as its etymology indicates, it refers to what we know with others, as a member of a group, formed by those associations to which we belong. Of course, many sources form one's conscience: upbringing, culture, education, and, in the case of physicians, one's profession.

That aspect of one's conscience that one's profession forms and upon which one relies as a practitioner amounts to the professional facet of one's conscience. Of course, this feature of one's conscience reflects the ethic internal to one's practice. As noted in 4.3, that ethic does not simply reiterate what morality might hold independently of one's formation as a member of the profession. Rather, in keeping with the internal ethic, one's professional conscience (if I may so speak) makes unique demands on one's conduct. Demands distinct from the morals one shares with others not of one's profession.

Consider capital punishment. For the sake of argument, concede both its justifiability and the incompatibility of participation in it with medical professionalism. Moreover, acknowledge the reasonableness of state officials' desire to employ medical technology to mitigate the distress of the condemned. Imagine a physician employed by a state's department of corrections. His principal charge would be the care of the prisoners as patients, entirely in keeping with his profession. As an employee (technically competent in such matters) of the department of corrections, state officials might understandably (albeit unreflectively) initially regard him as a candidate to administer the death penalty. However, given its incompatibility with his professional conscience and their recognition of the same (in part due to he and his peers having educated the wider public about the medical promise), they ought to forego asking him. Were such officials nonetheless to ask him for his cooperation, they ought to respect his due recourse to professional conscientious objection to participating (in violation of his solemn vow). By contrast (and I ask forbearance in the use of this example), were a veterinarian employed by the prison system (e.g., the prison incorporating a farm) she would presumably not have recourse to professional conscientious objection were she asked to administer the death penalty.[17] Indeed, given the incompatibility of killing and the medical profession, were correctional officials to seek competent assistance in imposing the death penalty, they might reasonably have recourse to veterinary medicine (for the training of executioners or for practitioners willing to administer it).

In sum, of physicians, professional medical autonomy requires governance of self and peers and education of the wider public concerning its implications, in particular as they bear on requests for a physician's assistance. Of patients and authorities, the healer's professional self-lawing especially asks that such appeals comport with the medical ethic. In the event of conflict between the professed ethic and a desire to employ medical technique, respect for professional autonomy calls for the development of alternatives (e.g., in the case of capital punishment, the training of competent, but not medical, executioners). The regard due such autonomy extends to honoring professional conscientious objection. Professional medical autonomy merits respect to the extent to which it is "for the benefit of the sick." Found at the beginning of the oath-proper, this phrase points toward a concluding reflection on medical professing, the *Oath*, and Hippocrates.

4.4 CONCLUSION: ONE OR MANY MEDICAL PROFESSIONS?

While agreement attends the basic norm—"as to diseases, practice two: help or do not harm" articulated in 4.3.2—disagreement does accompany this standard as we descend to particulars in answering salient questions attending it. What constitutes health, disease, help, and harm? As referencing what ought to be—the normative or prescriptive in contrast to the descriptive, what obtains here and now—my language indicates *a* (monolithic) professional medical ethic. This, however, does not reflect the actual diversity that accompanies different answers to these critical questions. Is appearance health such that elective cosmetic surgery counts as medical practice? Does routine infant male circumcision simply mutilate? Many such questions arise, some of much greater import than others. Answers diverge; hence, so do allied promises.

In chapter 3, we extensively considered the crucial dispute over killing one's patient or assisting her to kill herself as the Apollonian and

Asclepian accounts differ with the Hippocratic insight. As the contemporary accepted yet continuously controverted (within and without medicine) practice of elective abortion indicates and as the currently spreading legalization of PAS and euthanasia suggests, some clinicians regard killing or assisting in self-killing as compatible with medical practice. Clearly, such practitioners would not conscientiously take the oath-proper or anything along its lines. While most contemporary medical oaths remain entirely silent concerning killing, one notes an oath (allow it to remain nameless) incorporating language to the effect that a physician might have the "awesome responsibility" "to take a life." To the extent to which such dissensus results in actually disparate promises and practices, we might more accurately speak descriptively of medical professions, acknowledging (albeit not thereby endorsing) this assortment.

In the United States, the White Coat Ceremony serves as a witness to the variety of oaths. In this rite of passage, students matriculate into medical school. This ritual consists of oath-taking—and, of course, vesting with the physician's customary white coat. It instances a partial renaissance in solemn medical-promising. In 1993, Columbia University's medical college inaugurated this custom. Currently, the majority of US medical schools initiate students via this ceremony. While often modeled on the Hippocratic *Oath*, at different institutions students take diverse oaths, including ones fashioned by the individual student for him or herself.

This renewed practice of medical oath-taking indicates a shared sense among medical students and faculty of the solemnity attending medical practice. Caring for the ill involves one in deeply significant acts that merit the invocation of that which one holds sacred. Simply put, medicine involves professing—the *Oath's* legacy. That the vows taken vary, however, indicates a lack of consensus concerning the specifics to which medical practice commits one. Apparently, there is no longer one medical creed. Rather, one finds diverse pledges. Accordingly, one venerable source for designating medicine *a* profession has gone by the wayside. (Needless to say, one who regards medicine purely as a technique ought take no oath at all. He cannot lay claim to anything more than a nominal profession.)

Although medicine may no longer claim to be one profession, were a physician to have taken an oath, patients would naturally find this of interest. Moreover, a doctor would presumably want to share her view of her calling with those upon whom she practices. If oath-taking is to count for more than a mere gesture to a venerable past, then patients and the wider public ought to know to what did the practitioner pledge? (This fulfills one of the claims medical autonomy makes on those who profess, noted in 4.3.4. Namely, to educate the wider public as to the profession's commitments.) Aware of the variety of oaths taken, it might come to pass that patients would seek out physicians sharing a certain view of medicine. For instance, convinced of the soundness of the oath-proper, a patient might actively seek out a Hippocratic physician. Moreover, medical promising itself has promise. For example, given the opportunity, physicians, medical students, patients, and others who share an account of health and sickness will naturally form larger associations (e.g., practices, hospitals, and allied medical schools) comporting with their common vision. Indeed, the survival of the medical tradition associated with the *Oath* itself witnesses to the long-term viability of such developments. Of course, the *Oath* calls to mind Hippocrates.

For reasons noted in chapter 2, Hippocrates would not himself have taken the *Oath*, while he would have sworn the oath-proper (or its equivalent). Recall the blessing invoked by him who fulfills it:

> Now, to me making this oath fulfilled, and not breaking [it], may it be to share in life and art, being famous according to all men for all time; but [to me] transgressing and forswearing, the opposite of these.

As his fame evidences, Hippocrates more than kept his promise. For we speak well of him over two millennia after his passing from this bent world. While one barely discerns the remnants of the once majestic temples of Apollo, Asclepius, Hygeia, and Panacea, Hippocrates rightly remains famous for conceiving medicine as an exclusively therapeutic practice. This conception flowers in the medical profession: adroitly help the diseased; do not injure—especially, do not kill, sexually exploit, or gossip. Perennial, the oath-proper still illuminates the sure path of those exclusively devoted to mending. As argued, doctoring so understood remains eminently reasonable, viable, and attractive, well suited to the human condition. Therefore, let our conclusion echo Dante in his admiration of "that great Hippocrates whom nature made for the animals whom she loves most dearly" (*Purgatorio*, xxix, 137–8).[18]

Appendix

HIPPOCRATES' *OATH*— GREEK TEXT AND LITERAL ENGLISH TRANSLATION

What follows is an interlinear literal (and inelegant) translation of the *Oath*. Brackets indicate implied words. The translation sacrifices eloquence for accuracy. As much as possible, the English follows the actual Greek word order. The Greek—taken from the standard (and widely available) Hippocrates 1962—appears below the English translation. But for this translation's literalness, it follows the norm.

I swear by Apollo physician and Asclepius and Hygeia and Panacea
ὄμνυμι Ἀπόλλωνα ἰητρὸν καὶ Ἀσκληπιὸν καὶ Ὑγείαν καὶ Πανάκειαν

and by both all the gods and all [the goddesses], making [them my]
    witnesses,
καὶ θεοὺς πάντας τε καὶ πάσας, ἵστορας ποιεύμενος,

to fulfill according to my ability and judgment

ἐπιτελέα ποιήσειν κατὰ δύναμιν καὶ κρίσιν ἐμὴν

this oath and this contract;

ὅρκον τόνδε καὶ συγγραφὴν τήνδε·

to regard indeed my teacher in this art as equal to my parents,

ἡγήσεσθαι μὲν τὸν διδάξαντά με τὴν τέχνην ταύτην ἴσα γενέτῃσιν ἐμοῖς,

and of my livelihood to share [with him],

καὶ βίου κοινώσεσθαι,

and [to him] needing necessities to make [him] a share [of mine],

καὶ χρεῶν χρηΐζοντι μετάδοσιν ποιήσεσθαι,

and his male offspring to esteem as equal to [my] brothers,

καὶ γένος τὸ ἐξ αὐτοῦ ἀδελφοῖς ἴσον ἐπικρινεῖν ἄρρεσι,

and to teach [them] this art,

καὶ διδάξειν τὴν τέχνην ταύτην,

if they want to learn [it], without fee and contract,

ἢν χρηΐζωσι μανθάνειν, ἄνευ μισθοῦ καὶ συγγραφῆς,

of rule and lecture and all remaining teaching

παραγγελίης τε καὶ ἀκροήσιος καὶ τῆς λοίπης ἁπάσης μαθήσιος

I will make a share with my sons and those of my teacher,

μετάδοσιν ποιήσεσθαι υἱοῖς τε ἐμοῖς καὶ τοῖς τοῦ ἐμὲ διδάξαντος,

and with students contracted and oathed to the physician's law,

καὶ μαθητῆσι συγγεγραμμένοις τε καὶ ὠρκισμένοις νόμῳ ἰητρικῷ,

but to not one other.

ἄλλῳ δὲ οὐδενί.

Regimens I will use for the benefit of the sick

διαιτήμασί τε χρήσομαι ἐπ᾽ ὠφελείῃ καμνόντων

according to my ability and judgment,

κατὰ δύναμιν καὶ κρίσιν ἐμήν,

but [what is used] for harm and injustice I will keep away from [the sick].

ἐπὶ δηλήσει δὲ καὶ ἀδικίῃ εἴρξειν.

I will neither give a deadly drug to anyone, though having been asked,

οὐ δώσω δὲ οὐδὲ φάρμακον οὐδενὶ αἰτηθεὶς θανάσιμον,

nor will I lead the way to such counsel;

οὐδὲ ὑφηγήσομαι συμβουλίην τοιήνδε·

and, similarly, to a woman a destructive pessary I will not give.

ὁμοίως δὲ οὐδὲ γυναικὶ πεσσὸν φθόριον δώσω.

But purely and piously I will watch over my life and my art.

ἁγνῶς δὲ καὶ ὁσίως διατηρήσω βίον τὸν ἐμὸν καὶ τέχνην τὴν ἐμήν.

I will not cut, indeed, not even on those suffering from stone,

οὐ τεμέω δὲ οὐδὲ μὴν λιθιῶντας,

but I will give way to practicing men in this doing.

ἐκχωρήσω δὲ ἐργάτησιν ἀνδράσι πρήξιος τῆσδε.

Into as many houses as I enter, I will go into in order to benefit the sick,

ἐς οἰκίας δὲ ὁκόσας ἂν ἐσίω, ἐσελεύσομαι ἐπ ὠφελείῃ καμνόντων,

being free from all voluntary injustice and corruption,

ἐκτὸς ἐὼν πάσης ἀδικίης ἑκουσίης καὶ φθορίης,

especially sexual acts with the bodies of females and of males,

τῆς τε ἄλλης καὶ ἀφροδισίων ἔργων ἐπί τε γυναικείων σωμάτων καὶ
    ἀνδρῴων,

of free and of slaves.

ἐλευθέρων τε καὶ δούλων.

About whatever in therapy I see or hear,

ἃ δ' ἂν ἐν θεραπείῃ ἢ ἴδω ἢ ἀκούσω,

or also outside of therapy concerning the life of men,

ἢ καὶ ἄνευ θεραπείης κατὰ βίον ἀνθρώπων,

that ought never to be spoken out, I will be silent,

ἃ μὴ χρή ποτε ἐκλαλεῖσθαι ἔξω, σιγήσομαι,

holding such things not to be spoken.

ἄρρητα ἡγεύμενος εἶναι τὰ τοιαῦτα.

Now, to me making this oath fulfilled,

ὅρκον μὲν οὖν μοι τόνδε ἐπιτελέα ποιέοντι,

and not breaking [it],

καὶ μὴ συγχέοντι,

may it be to share in life and art,

εἴη ἐπαύρασθαι καὶ βίου καὶ τέχνης

being famous according to all men for all time;

δοξαζομένῳ παρὰ πᾶσιν ἀνθρώποις ἐς τὸν αἰεὶ χρόνον·

but [to me] transgressing and forswearing, the opposite of these.

παραβαίνοντι δὲ καὶ ἐπιορκέοντι, τἀναντία τούτων.

NOTES

CHAPTER 1

1. For a scholarly consideration of what we do know, see De Waele 1927.
2. Complicating matters further, in addition to the herald's staff, Hermes also bears a wand. In the older extant Greek stories about Hermes found, for example, in the *Homeric Hymn to Hermes* (dating to about 520 B.C. and called "Homeric" because it shares the same metrical pattern as writings attributed to Homer), we learn that Apollo gave Hermes "a marvelous wand with three gold branches." Apollo subsequently speaks of Hermes as the "bearer of the golden wand" (lines 530–540, Hyde 1998, 330). This magical wand must be distinguished from the *kērukeion* or herald's staff. It appears to be in terms of the magical wand that Hermes occupies a role particularly ill-suited to a physician, namely that of a *psychopompos* or soul-guide who conducts the dead to Hades. In the *Iliad*, Homer tells us that by means of his magical wand, Hermes "seals men's eyes in sleep or wakes them, just as he pleases" (*Iliad*, 24:342–3, Homer 1999a, 294). (This sealing of men's eyes in sleep includes, without being limited to, his role as soul-guide after death.) Thus, we see that true to form as a cunning god, Hermes carries both a magical wand and the herald's staff or caduceus, the latter of which becomes conflated with our quarry, Asclepius' staff.
3. I refer those interested in the whole history to Professor Friedlander's text, upon which I here rely: Friedlander 1992.
4. Friedlander 1992, ch. 7.
5. The French medical historian Jacques Jouanna brings to our attention a text from Hippocrates: "Another principle is the following: a disease arises because of similars, and, by being treated with similars, patients recover from such diseases" (Hippocrates 1995, 83). Jouanna writes, "Therapy by similars was already sufficiently known in the fifth century B.C. to have found expression in the theater with Sophocles: physicians: 'evacuate bitter bile with a bitter clyster'" (Jouanna 1999, 473–4). As Jouanna reminds us, while the Hippocratic corpus recognizes the occasional efficacy of

homeopathy, "Hippocratism is . . . founded on allopathy, or treatment by agents producing effects contrary to those of the disease (Jouanna 1999, 343)." As will be noted at greater length, the terms "allopathic" and "homeopathic" date to the 1800s.

6. To be precise, Hahnemann (the nineteenth-century advocate of homeopathy) proposes the Latin subjunctive *similia similibus curentur* or "let like be cured by like." Paracelsus, a Swiss-German Renaissance physician uses the Latin indicative *similia similibus curantur* or "like is cured by like." The two are, of course, not at odds; rather, the truth of the observation (stated by Paracelsus in the indicative) leads to the proposal (put in the subjunctive by Hahnemann).

7. Finding actual examples of effective homeopathic remedies (construed in the manner I call "specific") proves difficult. Zinc-gluconate, which produces runny noses in the healthy, may reduce the severity of the common cold. If so, it would be an instance of a homeopathic remedy. Hahnemann himself proposes cinchona (Peruvian bark), which in him produced malaria-like symptoms (perhaps due to an allergy of which he was unaware). The development in the healthy of such symptoms upon consumption of cinchona, however, does not seem to be the typical reaction. In the history of the use of cinchona as an anti-malarial, the effecting of such symptoms in one who consumed cinchona did not actually lead to its discovery or use as an anti-malarial. Rather, the indigenous Indians who lived at high altitudes (where malaria was not a problem) found that Peruvian bark—in Quechua called *kina*, from which we get "quinine"—reduced shivering due to extended exposure to cold temperature (which was a problem for them at high altitudes). (They steeped cinchona in hot water, drinking the resulting tea.) Subsequently, it appears that Europeans living at lower altitudes surmised that if the bark was efficacious against shivering, perhaps it might be helpful with the shivering attending malarial fever. It was. As we have come to learn, quinine, the active ingredient in the bark, both relaxes muscles (by which it ameliorates shivering) and disrupts the life-cycle of the parasite *Plasmodium* (by which it alleviates the malarial fever which the parasite causes).

8. One (first) finds *Homöopathie* in Hahnemann 2001, 461. He mints *Allopathie* (other than the disease)—in 1842 (Hahnemann 1982, 24). As Hahnemann proposes the term, "allopathy" means treating a disease with medicines "with no direct pathic relationship to the disease condition, [producing] symptoms neither similar nor opposite but completely heterogeneous" (Hahnemann 1982, 24). Of course, "allo" means "other than" in accordance with Hahnemann's use of the term. In contrast to his proposal, "allopathy" comes to mean "treating with opposites." Following the literal Greek meanings of "anti" and "enantio," Hahnemann proposes "antipathic" and "enantiopathic" to name approaches that employ medicines that produce symptoms opposite to those of the disease (Hahnemann 1982, p. 26).

9. Paul of Aegina, the seventh century A.D. medical encyclopedist writes of wounds called "telephian" in Book IV, section 46 of his *Medical Compendium*.

10. We find the relevant Hippocratic text in *Epidemics*, I, 11, literally translated as "concerning diseases, practice two: help or do not harm." W. H. S. Jones nicely translates it: "As to diseases make a habit of two things—to help, or at least to do no harm" (Hippocrates 1962, 164–5). The Greek infinitive (*askein*) translated with "practice"

connotes "practice skillfully." It suggests the development of finesse. As Albert Jonsen proposes, the better-known Latin phrase *primum non nocere* may have some association with Galen's commentary on the text from the *Epidemics* (Jonsen 1975, 40, note 1). Galen's Latin (found in Jonsen 1975) reads:"*oportet enim medicum imprimis aegrorum auxilio animum intendere sin minus ipsos tamen non laedere.*" A literal translation of Galen would read: "in the physician's mind it is necessary in the first place to seek to help the sick or at the least not to harm them." This does not amount to the pithy "*primum non nocere*," but one sees how it could become so by the twists and turns that reading, commentary, and human memory take.

11. Charles Bosk 2003, in his study of the socialization of erring surgical residents entitled *To Forgive and Remember*, records one way medicine treats erring practitioners. Namely, forgive the one who has committed an error, and remember the error so that he and others may learn to avoid it in the future.

12. Aristotle's father Nicomachus (after whom Aristotle named his son, to whom he dedicates the above-quoted work of ethics) was a physician in the court of the Macedonian King Amyntus II, whose grandson, Alexander the Great, Aristotle tutored. Had his father not died while Aristotle was a young man, Aristotle himself might have become a physician, following in his father's footsteps.

13. Aristotle's *Rhetoric*, I.1.1355b15–21, as translated—with slight modifications—by Garver 1994, 164.

14. Levine does not cite the source of Mead's comment. Perusal of the works by Mead cited in Levine's book does not reveal its origin. As Mead wrote the introduction to the book in which the quote occurs, it may be a personal communication to Levine.

CHAPTER 2

1. As Nails indicates, the Hippocrates of the *Protagoras* appears to be a nephew of Pericles I, belonging to the Alcmaeonid family (Nails 2002, 169–70).

2. Traditionally, fathers taught sons medicine. So, for example (as we will note in 2.2.2), Hippocrates' son-in-law and disciple Polybus (who himself wrote a treatise found in the Hippocratic corpus entitled *Nature of Man*) would have had to take the *Oath*. As Jouanna remarks: "Polybus . . . was obliged as Hippocrates' son-in-law and disciple to take the medical oath in order to enter the school of Cos, since he did not belong to the family by male descent" (Jouanna 1999, 51).

3. "The Asclepiads of Cos were well aware of their relatives on the neighboring island of Rhodes, where the medical tradition had died out" (Jouanna 1999, 48).

4. Translation adapted (slightly more literal) from the anonymous translation found in Aristophanes 1938, 880–1.

5. As a Greek, Hippocrates is entirely at home with oaths. Presumably, so also is the *Oath's* author. Certainly, he did not object to oaths or swearing by the gods. Nor is it probable that he belonged to an intellectual tradition hostile to oaths. Yet the medical historian Ludwig Edelstein proposes that the *Oath* has Pythagorean origins, while simultaneously noting that Pythagoras was famously reported to have forbade his

followers from swearing by the gods. As Edelstein notes, Pythagoras reportedly holds that in contrast to swearing by the gods, one "should rather make oneself the witness of one's own words." Edelstein goes on: "It is true, 'Pythagoras' tried to remedy the notorious Greek predilection for making oaths" (Edelstein 1967, 53). Were a Pythagorean to remedy this penchant by fashioning the most famous oath in history, he would prove a dubious disciple of the master. Moreover, the *Oath* closes with a blessing including "being well-regarded by all men for all time." The desire that one's reputation persist eternally does not comport with the Pythagorean doctrine of reincarnation.

6. One does not commonly swear by "all the goddesses." One notes that the extensive database kept by the University of Nottingham (http://www.nottingham.ac.uk/greatdatabase/brzoaths/public_html/database/index.php) contains only two other oaths that bring in "all the goddesses" as witnesses, one being comic and one being Alcibiades' (humorous) oath that he has slept with Socrates only in the way that one might sleep with one's older brother or father, found in the *Symposium*, 219c7–d2 (Plato 1925, 231). Of course, the comic often lampoons the most serious matters. The *Oath's* inclusion of "all the goddesses" indicates a vow of the most solemn significance. Perhaps, also, we here see an allusion to the otherwise unmentioned daughters of Asclepius, for example, Iaso, the goddess whose name means "healing."

7. *The Oxford Classical Dictionary*, 2d ed., s.v. "Apollo."

8. Notably, prior to Asclepius' cult coming to Athens, there is a reference to Athena Hygeia in Plutarch *Pericles* 13, as noted in *The Oxford Classical Dictionary*, 2nd ed., s.v. "*hygieia*." Thus, it seems as if Hygeia preceded her father's Athenian arrival.

9. In *Euthyphro* and *Apology* (Socrates' defense—the Greek word means a response to an accusation—in which he responds to a charge of impiety), Plato makes an extended argument that his teacher Socrates exemplifies piety. For piety consists of caring for something loved by the gods on behalf of the gods. Socrates piously ministers to the god-beloved Athenians by goading them on to attend to the best possible state of their souls. This therapeutic practice he defines as philosophizing.

10. See, for one recent example, Miles. He writes:

> "I will not give a drug that is deadly" follows the words "from injustice I will keep them" and thus seems to speak of the doctor's refusing to act at the behest of others who would commit an injustice in the public world. If this vow had been situated after "Into the houses I enter . . . while being far from all voluntary and destructive injustice," it seems more probable that it would have been a vow to refrain from using poison to end suffering during a clinical relationship. The physician-assassin damaged the trustworthiness of the entire profession, and the *Oath's* simple vow spoke to this fear. (Miles 2004, 74)

Miles rightly notes that the correct interpretation partially depends upon whom one pledges to keep "from injustice" (in the immediately preceding line in the *Oath*). Oddly, he suggests that the implied "them" refers not to the sick (the immediately preceding subjects on behalf of whom the juror "will use regimens" but, rather, those "in the public world" heretofore unmentioned. One need not search so far for that to which the oath-taker promises. The juror generally pledges not to use, but, rather, to keep the baneful and the unjust away from the aforementioned sick (*kamnontōn*). Following this generic promise, he then forswears a specific injury; namely, the giving of a deadly drug to a patient. Accordingly (and contrary to what Miles puzzlingly proposes), we do here encounter a clear, concise, and complete rejection of both giving one's patient a deadly drug if asked for it (either by the patient or by others) and counseling the same. By the *Oath*, the prospective physician rejects the act of giving a deadly drug to the sick as baneful, destructive, harmful, and unjust. As the juror acts to benefit the sick, he forswears both this maleficent act and the act of suggesting this maleficence.

11. E.g., "he" is in the nominative case; it indicates the role of a sentence's subject. "His" is in the genitive case; it indicates the role of possessor. "Him" is in the accusative; it points to the role of direct object.

12. As noted, *horkos* etymologically derives from the word for fence or boundary, *herkos*. Zeus serves as the god for both oaths and boundaries. Given the privilege of entering the house, the *Oath* binds its taker not to violate the boundary. Taking the *Oath* renders one worthy of the trust needed to cross the threshold.

CHAPTER 3

1. As is customary, "euthanasia" refers to voluntary active euthanasia, while PAS refers to physician-assisted suicide. Some speak of the latter as "physician-assisted death" or "physician aid in dying." These phrases do not prove helpful. For they do not adequately distinguish the relevant practice from many others that involve a physician's help at the end of one's life. Currently, both practices involve a competent terminally ill patient (whose prognosis indicates death within six months) requesting either that her physician kill her by lethal injection (in the case of euthanasia) or write her a prescription for a lethal drug that she herself takes (PAS).

2. Needless to say, the doctor, physician, healer, or mender always cares, but may not always cure. As the French proverb (whose origins remain obscure) would have it, the role of the doctor is *"guérir quelquefois, soulager souvent, consoler toujours,"* or "to cure sometimes, to relieve often, to console always."

3. Charles Henry Sanson spoke these words in the summer of 1766 to the twenty-something Chevalier de la Barre prior to decapitating him by sword. He did so in response to the Chevalier's bantering with him about Sanson's involvement (approximately two months previously) in the famously botched, exceptionally grisly execution of Comte Thomas Arthur de Lally-Tollendall (on May 6, 1766). Sanson suggested that the Comte's lack of composure led to the fiasco. The Chevalier was put to death standing up (on July 1, 1766), as he considered kneeling fit for a criminal, which he emphatically did not regard himself. Reputedly, the Chevalier showed such mental fortitude and Sanson's stroke was so powerfully, swiftly, and sharply delivered that the young man's head momentarily remained atop his still-standing corpse before

both toppled to the ground in front of an amazed assemblage (Sanson 1881, 116–7). Clearly, de la Barre possessed the requisite firmness.

4. For example, in 1699 Madame Angeline-Nicole Tiquet and the commoner Jacques Moura were both found guilty of attempting to murder her husband, Monsieur Tiquet. Moura, a hotel porter, was condemned to die by hanging, Madame Tiquet to be decapitated by sword. One notes, as was sometimes the case with decapitations by sword, that Moura in this instance seems to have suffered the less gruesome fate. After the hanging of Moura, the executioner Charles Sanson de Longval (the first of seven generations of Sanson executioners and the great-grandfather of the above noted Charles Henry Sanson) took three increasingly grisly strokes to sever the neck of the famously beautiful Madame. Again, decapitation by sword was not necessarily a coup de grâce. In proposing the guillotine, the surgeon Louis recalls (in his *Avis motivé sur le mode de décollation*) the (previously noted) dreadful execution of Comte Thomas Arthur de Lally-Tollendall of 1766:

> The executioner [the great-grandson of Charles Sanson de Longval] struck him on the back of the neck. The blow did not separate the head from the body, nor could it have done. Nothing now prevented the body from falling. It toppled forward, and the head was finally separated from the body by four or five sabre blows. This hacking [*bacherie*], if we may use the term, was witnessed with horror" (Arasse 1989, 186; original French edition, Arasse 1987, 209).

5. "*Il y a des hommes malheureux; Christophe Colomb ne peut attacher son nom à sa découverte; Guillotin ne peut détacher le sien de son invention*" (Hugo 1976, 299).

6. Pellet quotes the original French source, the newspaper *Les Actes des Apôtres* 1, no. 10: 156–7.

7. "*Avec ma machine, je vous fais sauter la tête en un clin d'œil et sans que vous éprouviez la moindre douleur.*"

8. In *Laws* Plato notably insists upon death for the physician who attempts to poison while subjecting a layman to punishment or fine as determined by the court. He regards the physician's offence as especially egregious, requiring the gravest penalty (Plato 1961, 933d4–5, 1484).

9. I thank Thomas Marcus Cavanaugh, who graciously brought this remarkable text to my attention as a dramatic illustration of the import of physicians' refraining from killing their patients.

10. The following is representative of the widely acknowledged evidence that suicidal individuals stand ambivalently toward their self-induced deaths:

> It is estimated that only one out of ten suicide attempts results in death, a figure that tends to confirm the view that suicidal individuals are conflicted about dying. Similarly, studies of the subsequent mortality rates of survivors show that only about 1 percent of all survivors kill themselves within one year. Thus intervention—even if it is short-term and circumscribed—seems warranted and desirable. (Hendin 1995, 237)

For reflection upon the confusion caused among the more generally suicidal by physician involvement in the killing of a patient, see Hendin 1997.

11. The psychiatrist Herbert Hendin, MD, an authority concerning suicide in the United States, notes:

> If the Dutch experience teaches us anything it is that euthanasia brings out the worst rather than the best in medicine. . . . Instead of expanding patient's choices, euthanasia becomes a seemingly simple solution for a myriad of problems. Pressure for improved palliative care appears to have evaporated in the Netherlands. Discussion of care for those who are terminally ill is dominated by how and when to extend euthanasia to increasing groups of patients. (Hendin 1997, 214)

Innovation depends on dissatisfaction with the status quo. If euthanizing one's patient resolves his condition, who needs or would reasonably want to develop alternatives?

12. To mention one more popularly available example, in *David and Goliath* Malcolm Gladwell recounts the story of the physician Emil "Jay" Freireich, who pioneered the treatment of children suffering from leukemia, originally a dreadful death sentence (Gladwell 2013, 125–64). Now, the prognosis for a child with leukemia is a better than likely chance of survival. Were the killing of children suffering from leukemia a therapeutic option at the time of Freireich's innovations, one reasonably doubts that the remarkable advancements he and his colleagues achieved would have come about as readily (not that they were easily arrived at). Therapeutic progress in the treatment of a specific disease will diminish as and, presumably, to the very extent to which physicians and society more generally come to regard the killing of a patient suffering from that illness as a therapy.

13. For a description of an actual instance, see the case Ira Byock, MD (a hospice physician expert in palliation) presents (Byock 1997, 209–16). One typically need not resort to terminal sedation to comfort a patient adequately at the end of life. As Byock notes, however, there remain instances in which one can relieve distress at agonal pain only by sedation. For an extensive treatment of the overarching account (referred to as double-effect reasoning) distinguishing the ethical character of terminal sedation from PAS and euthanasia, see Cavanaugh 2006.

14. For a helpful consideration of the distinction within the law as found in the U.K and in the United States, see Keown 2002, 22–30. Also, see the majority and concurring opinions in *Washington v. Glucksberg* 521 U.S. 702 (1997) and *Vacco v. Quill*, 521 U.S., 793 (1997) in which the US Supreme Court acknowledges the tenability of a state distinguishing between (legal) terminal sedation and (illegal) PAS. For a treatment of the ethical account underlying the public policy by which legislators distinguish terminal sedation from PAS and euthanasia, see Cavanaugh 2006, especially 183–90.

CHAPTER 4

1. In my usage I do not distinguish a vow from an oath. However, some thinkers (aptly) distinguish a vow by which one promises to a deity from an oath by which one

promises to fellow mortals. In Latin, a vow is a *votum*, from the verb *voveo*, meaning "to promise sacredly"; an oath is a *juramentum*, from the verb *juro*, meaning "to swear." In keeping with this distinction, one may invoke the divine as a witness to an oath, but the promise is to mortals. For an interesting and extensive discussion of the difference between a vow and an oath, see Thomas Aquinas, *Summa theologiae*, IIaIIae, questions 88 and 89: Aquinas 1962, 1452–72. The Ancient Greeks do not appear to make this distinction, perhaps because in some sense for them one always (at least partially) swears to the gods and not simply by them.

2. The quote at the end of this passage belongs to the physician Asclepiades of Bithynia—modern-day Turkey—who lived circa 124—40 B.C. and furthered the establishment of Greek medicine in Rome.

3. One finds the Latin original in line 5 of the preface of *Compositiones* (Largus 1983, 2). Scribonius seems to have originally been from Sicily, since he knows the rare Sicilian trefoil, an indigenous plant that serves as a remedy for snakebite. He first records its Latin name (*trifolium acutum*, Largus 1983, 94), while also knowing the Greek (*oxytriphyllon* Largus 1983, 163) as would an educated Sicilian of his time (see Hanson 2010, 498). Moreover, the locally famous Sicilian physician Apuleius Celsus, from the city of Centuripae (present-day Centuripe, Sicily), taught him medicine suggesting Scribonius' own origins.

4. Here is Aulus Cornelius Celsus: *"Et per hos quidem maxime viros salutaris ista nobis professio increvit."* "And through these men mostly this salutary profession of ours has grown up" (Celsus 1935, 6, author's translation). Celsus says this after having mentioned, among others, Asclepius and Hippocrates. Celsus' reference to medicine as a profession serves in Lewis and Short's *A Latin Dictionary* to illustrate *professio* when applied to a "business or profession which one publicly avows," s.v. *"professio."* Celsus' eloquent Latin in the Renaissance earned him the sobriquet *Cicero medicorum*, "Cicero of the physicians."

5. A nun differs from a sister in part due to a difference in their vows. A nun takes solemn vows; a sister, simple. With respect to the vow of poverty, for example, the nun's solemn vow requires her to forego all ownership of property; by contrast, the sister's simple vow does not oblige her to forgo all such ownership.

6. Vanberg (2008) provides reasons for thinking that we keep a promise more for the very sake of keeping the promise than for avoiding the disappointment that others who placed trust in us would experience were we to break the promise.

7. I use the phrase "other things being equal" to acknowledge that a promise needs, e.g., not to be rash, frivolous, or unjust. If I unjustly vow, e.g., to harm an innocent, other things are not equal. Thus, while my so swearing might explain my act of harming the innocent, it certainly does not justify it.

8. In keeping with this ancient usage, contemporary medical ethics customarily considers a patient as autonomous. See the entry in Liddell and Scott's *An Intermediate Greek-English Lexicon*, 7th ed., s.v. *"autonomos."*

9. I recommend and rely on—but do not do justice to—Alasdair MacIntyre's magisterial treatment of practices and the goods internal and external to them (MacIntyre, 1984, 181–203).

10. Author's translation of Aquinas' Latin: "*quaedam rationis ordinatio ad bonum commune, ab eo qui curam communitatis habet, promulgata,*" *Summa theologiae*, IaIIae, q.90, a.4, corpus; Aquinas 1962, 942.

11. A study in its own right, the distinction between common goods and private goods admits of differences of degree. Goods exist on a spectrum. On one end we find justice, which is entirely common; on the other, an apple, which is completely private. Perhaps because they tend to be physical and of immediate, obvious, and vital interest to us, we apprehend private goods more readily. To enjoy the apple one eats it. One's consumption of it necessarily excludes others from its use. Hence, it instances a private good. Justice, by contrast, cannot be enjoyed alone. One's enjoyment of justice necessarily involves others' enjoyment of it rather than necessarily excluding them. Justice and the apple stand at the extremes in the spectrum of common and private goods. A park, playing court, Olympic-sized pool, bridge, road, school, college, university, hospital, place of worship, library, or museum (to name a few examples) exists in between these extremes. As a finite good, one's enjoyment of, e.g., a park can diminish with the number of people enjoying it at any given time. However, it has aspects of a common good (as do the other noted examples) insofar as one's enjoyment of it does not exhaust it (and, thereby, necessarily exclude others, as would one's use of an entirely private good). However, one's utilizing of the park does not necessarily include others, as would a thoroughly common good.

12. Why distinguish diverse ways of employing reason at all? Why not simply regard reason as one without distinction? Briefly, when one employs reason to know (speculatively), one evaluates the intellect using the world as the standard of correctness. By contrast, when one employs reason to make the world a certain way (practically), one assesses the world using what the agent had in mind as the norm determining success. Philosophers sometimes speak of these different standards of evaluation or success as the diverse "directions of fit" found in reason employed speculatively or practically. Of course, truth instances success for reason. Among others, Aquinas defines truth as an adequacy between mind and the world. In the case of speculative truth, world judges mind; in practical, mind judges world. I know what water is when my concept of water adequates to what water is in the world. The world makes the mind to be a certain way. This is speculative truth. By contrast, practical knowledge makes the world to be a certain way. Hence, practical truth occurs when the water in the glass adequates to what I planned to do—to fill a glass with water. This is practical truth. In part because the direction of fit of reason successfully employed speculatively (speculative truth) differs from that of reason successfully employed practically (practical truth), one distinguishes the two uses of reason.

13. In Aquinas' Latin, "*bonum est faciendum et prosequendum et malum vitandum*" (*Summa theologiae*, IaIIae, q. 94 a. 2; 1962, 955). Aquinas refers to this most basic rule of reason employed practically as the first precept of the natural law.

14. By contrast, the first principle of reason employed speculatively is not a law subject to violation; it expresses how things are, not how they ought to be.

15. The *Oath* approximates this axiom in the passage (addressed in 2.2.3.1) reading: "Regimens I will use for the benefit of the sick according to my ability and judgment; but [what is used] for harm and injustice I will keep away from [the sick]."

16. Author's translation of: *"Alle Dinge sind Gift, und nichts ohne Gift, allein die Dosis macht dass ein Ding kein Gift ist"* (Paracelsus 1915, 25).

17. By this example I do not wish to denigrate the dignity of the condemned person by equating him to an animal. I want solely to note that the medical profession excludes the act of deliberate killing, independently of the morality of the killing so excluded. Veterinary medicine differs in this respect. For its internal code does not exclude executing a person—assuming that act can at times be done justly. Needless to say, a veterinarian may object (as may anyone) to administering the death penalty upon grounds other than its incompatibility with her profession.

18. Author's translation of *"quel sommo Ipocrate che natura/ A li animali fè ch' ell' ha più cari"* (Alighieri 1933, 601).

REFERENCES

Ainsworth, W. H. 1863. "Seven Generations of Executioners." *New Monthly Magazine* 127(57): 253–74.

Alighieri, D. 1933. *La divina commedia*. Edited by C. H. Grandgent. Boston: Heath.

Aquinas. 1962. *Summa theologiae*. Roma: Editiones Paulinae.

Arasse, D. 1987. *La guillotine et l'imaginaire de la terreur*. Paris: Flammarion.

Arasse, D. 1989. *The Guillotine and the Terror*. Translated by C. Miller. London: Penguin.

Aristophanes. 1938. *The Complete Greek Drama*. Vol. 2. Edited by W. J. Oates and E. O'Neill. New York: Random House.

Aristophanes. 2002. *Wealth/Plutus*. Edited and translated by J. Henderson. Cambridge, MA: Harvard University Press.

Aristotle. 1941. *The Basic Works of Aristotle*. Edited by R. McKeon. New York: Random House.

Aristotle. 1989. *Metaphysics*. Translated by H. Tredennick. Cambridge, MA: Harvard University Press.

Aristotle. 1990a. *Nicomachean Ethics*. Vol. 1. Translated by H. Rackham. Cambridge, MA: Harvard University Press.

Aristotle. 1990b. Politics. Translated by H. Rackham. Cambridge, MA: Harvard University Press.

Bosk, C. 2003. *To Forgive and Remember: Managing Medical Failure*. 2nd ed. Chicago: University of Chicago Press.

Byock, I. 1997. *Dying Well: Prospects for Growth at the End of Life*. New York: Riverhead.

Cavanaugh, T. A. 2006. *Double-Effect Reasoning: Doing Good and Avoiding Evil*. Oxford: Clarendon Press.

Celsus. 1935. *De medicina*. Vol. 1, books 1–4. With an English translation by W. G. Spencer. Cambridge, MA: Harvard University Press.

Chaucer, G. 2005. *The Canterbury Tales*. Edited by J. Mann. London: Penguin.

Cohen, M. R. 1999. *Medication Errors*. Washington, DC: American Pharmaceutical Association.

Croker, J. W. 1853. *History of the Guillotine*. London: John Murray.

De Waele, F. J. M. 1927. *The Magic Staff or Rod in Graeco-Italian Antiquity*. Ghent: Erasmus.

Edelstein, L. 1967. *Ancient Medicine: Selected Papers of Ludwig Edelstein*. Edited by O. Temkin and C. L. Temkin, 3–63. Baltimore: The Johns Hopkins University Press.

Fletcher, J. 2012. *Performing Oaths in Classical Greek Drama*. New York: Cambridge University Press.

Fontenrose, J. 1978. *The Delphic Oracle: Its Responses and Operations with a Catalogue of Responses*. Berkeley: University of California Press.

Friedlander, W. J. 1992. *The Golden Wand of Medicine: A History of the Caduceus Symbol in Medicine*. Westport: Greenwood Press.

Garver, E. 1994. *Aristotle's Rhetoric: An Art of Character*. Chicago: University of Chicago Press.

Gladwell, M. 2013. *David and Goliath: Underdogs, Misfits, and the Art of Battling Giants*. New York: Little, Brown.

Guillotin, J-I. 1844. *Chambers's Edinburgh Journal* 1(14): 218–21.

Hahnemann, S. 1982. *Organon of Medicine*. Translated by J. Künzu, A. Naudé, and P. Pendleton. Los Angeles: J. P. Tarcher.

Hahnemann, S. 2001. *Gesammelte kleine Schriften*. Edited by J. Schmidt and D. Kaiser. Heidelberg: K. F. Haug.

Hamilton, J. S. 1986. Scribonius Largus on the Medical Profession. *Bulletin of the History of Medicine* 60: 209–16.

Hanson, A. 2010. Roman Medicine. In *A Companion to the Roman Empire*. Edited by D. Potter, 492–523. Oxford: Wiley-Blackwell.

Hendin, H. 1995. *Suicide in America*. New York: W. W. Norton.

Hendin, H. 1997. *Seduced by Death: Doctors, Patients, and the Dutch Cure*. New York: W. W. Norton.

Hickie, W. J. 1853. *The Comedies of Aristophanes*. Vol. 1. London: Bohn.

Hippocrates. 1962. *Epidemics I and III, Oath*. Vol. 1. Translated by W. H. S. Jones. Cambridge, MA: Harvard University Press.

Hippocrates. 1995. *Places in Man*. Translated by P. Potter. Cambridge, MA: Harvard University Press.

Hobbes, T. 1998. *Leviathan*. Edited by J. C. A. Gaskin. Oxford: Oxford University Press.

Homer. 1999a. *Iliad*. Translated by S. Butler. New York: Dover.

Homer. 1999b. *Iliad*. Vol. 1, books 1–12. Translated by A. T. Murray, revised by W. F. Wyatt. Cambridge, MA: Harvard University Press.

Hugo, V. 1976. *Littérature et philosophie mêlées*. Vol. 1. Edited by A. R. W. James. Paris: Klincksieck.

Hyde, L. 1998. *Trickster Makes This World*. New York: Farrar, Straus, and Giroux.

Jonsen, A. 1975. Do No Harm: Axiom of Medical Ethics. In *Philosophical Medical Ethics: Its Nature and Significance*. Edited by S. Spicker and H. T. Engelhardt, 27–41. Boston: D. Reidel.

Jonsen, A. 1990. *The New Medicine and the Old Ethics*. Cambridge, MA: Harvard University Press.

Jouanna, J. 1999. *Hippocrates*. Translated by M. B. DeBevoise. Baltimore: Johns Hopkins University Press.

Jouanna, J. 2012. *Greek Medicine from Hippocrates to Galen: Selected Papers.* Edited by P. van der Eijk and translated by N. Allies. Boston: Brill.

Keown, J. 2002. *Euthanasia, Ethics and Public Policy: An Argument against Legalisation.* Cambridge, UK: Cambridge University Press.

Kershaw, A. 1993. *A History of the Guillotine.* New York: Barnes and Noble.

Largus, S. 1983. *Scribonii Largi compositiones.* Edited by S. Sconocchia. Leipzig: Teubner.

Lauritzen, P. 2013. *The Ethics of Torture: Professional Responsibility in an Age of Terror.* Washington, DC: Georgetown University Press.

Levine, M. 1972. *Psychiatry and Ethics.* New York: Braziller.

MacIntyre, A. 1984. *After Virtue.* 2nd ed. Notre Dame: University of Notre Dame Press.

Miles, S. 2004. *The Hippocratic Oath and the Ethics of Medicine.* New York: Oxford University Press.

Miles, S. 2006. *Oath Betrayed: Torture, Medical Complicity, and the War on Terror.* New York: Random House.

Nails, D. 2002. *The People of Plato: A Prosopography of Plato and Other Socratics.* Indianapolis: Hackett.

N. C. 2009. *North Carolina Department of Corrections v. North Carolina Medical Board.* 675 S. E. 2d.

Paracelsus. 1915. *Sieben Defensiones.* Edited by K. Sudhoff. Leipzig: Barth.

Parke, H. W., and D. E. W. Wormell. 1961. *The Delphic Oracle.* Vol. 2. Oxford: Basil Blackwell.

Pellet, M. 1873. *Un journal royaliste en 1789: Les actes des apôtres (1789–1791).* Paris: Armand Le Chevalier.

Plato. 1925. *Plato: Lysis, Symposium, Gorgias.* With an English translation by W. R. M. Lamb. Cambridge, MA: Harvard University Press.

Plato. 1961. *The Collected Dialogues of Plato.* Edited by E. Hamilton and H. Cairns. Princeton: Princeton University Press.

Plescia, J. 1970. *The Oath and Perjury in Ancient Greece.* Tallahassee: Florida State University Press.

Plutarch. 1992. *Plutarch's Lives: The Lives of the Noble Grecians and Romans.* Translated by J. Dryden, revised by A. H. Clough. New York: Modern Library.

Sanson, H. 1881. *Memoirs of the Sansons: Seven Generations of Executioners, 1688–1847.* London: Chatto and Windus.

Vanberg, C. 2008. "Why Do People Keep Their Promises? An Experimental Test of Two Explanations." *Econometrica* 76(6): 1467–80.

Weiner, D. B. 1972. "The Real Doctor Guillotin." *Journal of the American Medical Association* 220(1): 85–9.

Wickkiser, B. L. 2008. *Asklepios, Medicine, and the Politics of Healing in Fifth-Century Greece: Between Craft and Cult.* Baltimore: Johns Hopkins University Press.

INDEX